FOOD HYGIENE FOR FOOD HANDLERS

A PRIMARY COURSE IN FOOD HYGIENE FOR FOOD WORKERS

by Cathal Kearney

Sponsored by

ALTRO

– FLOORING AND WALLING SPECIALIST –

and its Irish distributors

BROOKS THOMAS AND WESTILE

Published by:

Environmental Health Officers' Association

FOOD HYGIENE FOR FOOD HANDLERS

A Primary Course in Food Handling for Food Workers

Written by:
Cathal Kearney.

Published by:
Environmental Health Officers' Association,
PO Box 29,
Wicklow Town,
County Wicklow,
Republic of Ireland.

First Edition.

Edited by:
WordSmith PR & Editorial Services.

Design & Layout:
KMD Design.

Printed by:
Berry Print Group,
Golf Road,
Westport,
Co. Mayo.

ISBN: 0-9537955-0-0

Page

Acknowledgements
Photographs on pages 6 and 8 reproduced courtesy of European Commission Audio Visual Library and the photograph on page 70 reproduced courtesy of Science Footage Ltd. (UK).

Introduction

Having worked as an Environmental Health Officer for over twenty years, I have seen the enormous changes in the expectation of consumers in relation to the quality and safety of the food that they eat. This has been influenced by many factors including almost daily food scares and a recognition that poor food hygiene can result in serious illness. Here in Ireland, we have earned a good reputation for wholesome food production and we need to build on this even further. There has been a recognition at all levels from consumer to legislators that we need to be able to assure clean safe food for ourselves and our families.

The need for increased diligence has been forced upon us also by the recognition of new super bugs such as E-coli H0157 and Listeria. We still have a lot to learn about how these bugs infect food and cause illness. The European Union and our own Government have shown a commitment to improve the safety of our food through recent more stringent legislation, employment of additional food control staff, and the very welcome establishment of the Food Safety Authority of Ireland.

Since 1998 all food workers here in Ireland must be suitably trained in good food hygiene practices and all food businesses must establish a Hazard Analysis Critical Control Point (HACCP) or similar type food safety system within their food businesses. These requirements pose an immense challenge to the food industry and to people like myself as representatives of the consumer in having a responsibility for overseeing food premises.

This book is part of an effort to try to meet these new challenges. I set out to write the book in plain, simple language and in as uncomplicated a manner as possible. I hope that it can be a means of assisting food staff who are undertaking a primary course in Food Hygiene as well as being a brief reference book for people entering the food business for the first time. As many food poisoning incidents still occur within the home, I hope that it will also be of benefit for all who prepare food whether in commercial premises or not. So as to keep the book reasonably readable as well as short, some topics are dealt with in a summary manner only.

Proceeds from the sale of this book are returned to the Environmental Health Officer's Association for the support and further development of food hygiene training and health promotion.

We gratefully acknowledge the support of Altro Ltd and its distributors for their substantial sponsorship towards the production and printing of this book.

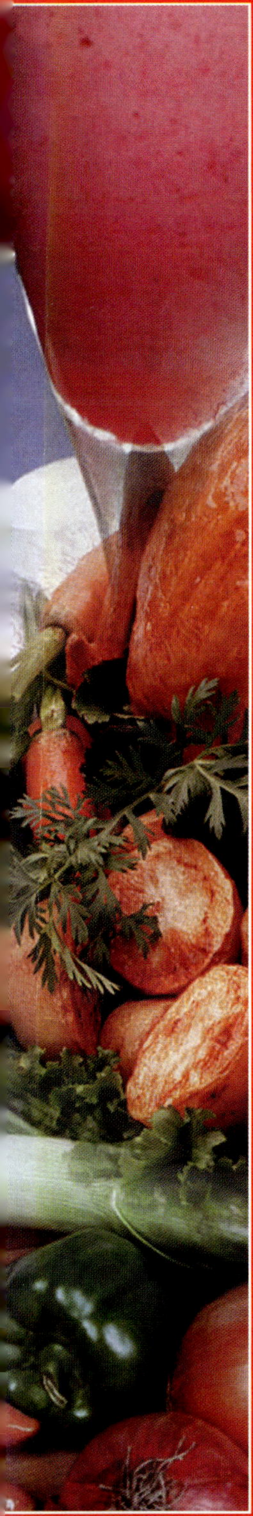

CHAPTER 1

WHY IS FOOD HYGIENE IMPORTANT?

The practice of good food hygiene not only safeguards the health of consumers but it also makes good business sense. Businesses that fail to recognise this reality are losing touch with the requirements of their customers.

A food handler, or the proprietor of a food business, must be concerned with food hygiene for a number of critical reasons:

1. Prevention of Food Poisoning

Food prepared in an unhygienic manner or under unhygienic conditions may cause those who consume it to become very ill which, in very severe cases, can result in death. Anyone who has suffered food poisoning knows that it is not usually just an "upset tummy" that sorts itself out in a few hours - it can result in a serious illness for up to a week and sometimes even longer.

The human misery caused by food poisoning or food-borne disease can be extremely distressing in terms of pain and discomfort. While death from food poisoning is, thankfully, a rare occurrence, the thought that a person's death might have resulted from your lack of knowledge or lack of care doesn't bear thinking about. Considering that standards of food hygiene have improved so much, it may seem odd that food poisoning is all too common but there is an explanation for this. As recently as 25 years ago, many more people in Ireland ate food which was home-grown or produced locally and which was invariably prepared in people's own homes, so that if food poisoning resulted, only a few people were affected. Today most of our food is produced in large quantities and often transported thousands of kilometres before reaching the local supermarket or restaurant.

Many now eat away from home and most people buy convenience foods that are already substantially prepared. So instead of just a few people being affected in the production 25 years ago, today's food may have been through ten different companies or handlers before reaching the consumer. This provides more opportunity for the food to be badly stored or handled. Moreover, instead of the fresh local products of the past, we now have food which keeps longer due to processing, thereby allowing more time for the food to become contaminated or support the growth of germs. Instead of four or five people at home being affected, hundreds can be affected at a local function.

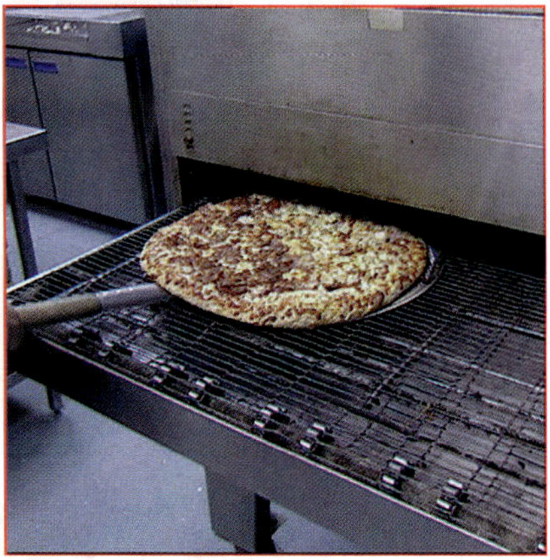

All food must be cooked to a temperature above 74°C to prevent harmful bacteria surviving the cooking process.

The toll of human suffering caused by food poisoning cannot be measured in financial terms. Nonetheless there is an enormous financial cost too when we remember that a lot of work days are lost through food poisoning. It is difficult to measure just how much financial loss is involved as food poisoning is considerably under-reported.

The good news is, of course, that food poisoning can be prevented.

Good Hygiene - Good Business

The public is now more conscious of good food hygiene than at any time in the past. All food workers are expected to practise good food hygiene in clean, hygienic premises. If the proprietor fails to realise this it does not augur well for the future of the business. Failure to invest human and financial resources in maintaining a high standard in the premises results in customers developing a poor image of the business. Customers then frequent the premises less, and so a decline in trading seems to justify the need for the proprietor to save resources and cut back in standards even further. And so the decline in trade continues.

On the other hand I have seen many food premises that were in very poor condition, with poor trade, being transformed in every sense following a decision to invest in modernisation with a strong emphasis on food hygiene. For example, a baker who employed two people in a premises that was badly run down, was forced to decide whether to abandon the business or invest in improvements following a Health Board prosecution (the voluntary way is so much easier!).

This baker obtained a loan to build a new bakery to a good standard. Within a year he had increased his profit through additional sales to the point where he needed to employ twice as many staff and where his profits were double what he previously realised ... and that was after he had deducted repayments for the loan.

Good food hygiene is a very saleable product and in a food business is as necessary as good management. You have only to look around at the standard of businesses which are obviously doing well to see that truth of that statement.

A premises that is operated in an hygienic manner is also conducive to good working conditions for staff and enables them to be justly proud of their workplace.

Reputation

If somebody became ill due to eating contaminated food from your premises your business would soon gain a bad reputation. Even worse, you could be taken to court by the Health Board and by the person or people who became ill. As a result, your business and livelihood could be ruined. It has happened in the past and is likely to happen again in the future. The best way to ensure that it doesn't happen is to practise good hygiene.

Legal responsibility

The Food Hygiene Regulations and the Hygiene of Foodstuffs Regulations that are in force in Ireland place a legal responsibility on each food worker to practice good food hygiene. This responsibility can be discharged only when you know what good food hygiene entails. If your washing machine broke down and you called a service engineer to fix it, you would expect that person to know how the machine works. Just as you are entitled to

Customers are entitled to be served good quality, safe food on your premises.

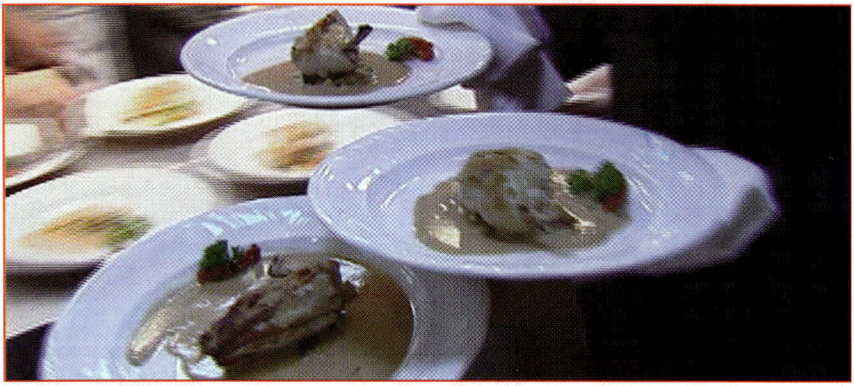

expect the service engineer to do the work you are paying for, so a customer consuming food in or from your premises is also entitled to expect you to know how to prepare food hygienically and always to put this knowledge into practice.

A food handler who prepares or handles food un-hygienically can be prosecuted personally by the Health Board under criminal law. Naturally this is the last course of action that anybody wants to pursue. Co-operation rather than conflict is the preferred relationship between food businesses and the statutory authorities who are given the task of supervising standards.

Employment -Tourism - Trust

Ireland has deservedly gained a reputation for being a source of good quality, natural, wholesome food ... a far cry from the "dirty Irish" which was once all too prevalent. It is important for all of us to build on our new image. Environmental controls, good animal husbandry and a commitment to good food hygiene will enhance this reputation further. This enhancement will increase employment in such areas as food processing and tourism and result in the whole community, including the food worker, having a better standard of living.

Sometimes I feel that we often behave in a certain manner because we are afraid of getting caught doing the wrong thing. I would like to think that we practise good hygiene because we know that it is the right thing to do. If food workers handle soiled toilet paper and fail to wash their hands before handling food, they have broken the trust which the customer has placed in them and in the premises where they work. The food is then served to the customer contaminated with the germs from the toilet paper. To put it another way, would you, as a customer, like to think that the slice of cooked turkey you bought in the shop was handled in the same manner as if it had been touched with soiled toilet paper?.

You can't see the germs but surely you trusted the food worker who sliced the meat for you?

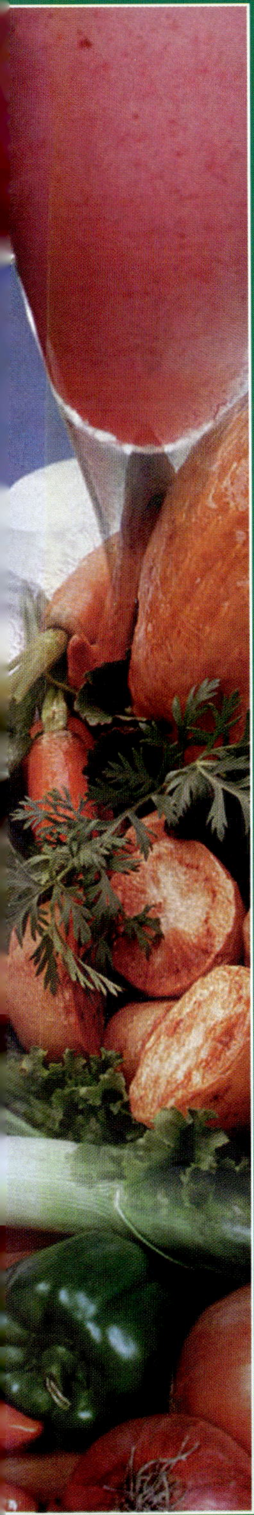

2

CHAPTER 2

FOOD CONTAMINATION

Food can become contaminated in a number of different ways. Knowing how this happens and how to control the levels of contamination can enable us to take precautions that are critical to the safety of food we produce.

Food Contamination

We now know why food hygiene is important. Remember that our greatest concern is that poor food hygiene can lead to people who consume contaminated food becoming ill. We commonly use the name "germ" to describe tiny creatures that cause us harm. Almost all food poisoning is caused by contamination with certain "germs" called bacteria. But food can also be contaminated with other small organisms such as moulds, yeast, fungi, viruses and parasites. Some of these organisms cause the food to become spoiled - for example, mouldy bread. In addition, food can also be contaminated by foreign bodies or chemicals. Since contamination with bacteria is the most important concern for us, we will deal with this form of contamination first.

Bacterial Contamination

So as to prevent food poisoning caused by bacteria we need to know: where bacteria are to be found, whether or not they are dangerous, how do they get on to our food, and how they grow on food? With such knowledge we are better equipped to try to prevent food becoming contaminated in the first place or at least prevent the bacteria from growing on our food.

What are bacteria?

All bacteria have a few common traits that are important to remember:

- Like all living entities bacteria grow, reproduce, eat, expel waste products and die.
- They cannot move from place to place by themselves: they must be carried on food, hands, clothes, or even by air currents.
- Because they are so small, they can only be seen using a microscope and cannot be seen with the naked eye. So from a practical viewpoint, as far as food hygiene is concerned, they can be considered invisible.
- Given ideal conditions for growth, such as a favourable temperature, they can multiply on food at an alarming rate, doubling in numbers every twenty minutes or so.

Where are bacteria found?

Bacteria can be found almost anywhere - in the soil, in water, in the air, on foods, on work-tops and cloths, as well as in and on our bodies. In fact it is easier to mention some of the few places where they are not found - in sterile liquids, for example, the drip you would see connected to a patient in a hospital. Again as far as food hygiene is concerned, we can simply say that bacteria are found everywhere.

Are bacteria harmful?

Only a small number of bacteria cause illness or disease and these are called "pathogenic" bacteria. Most bacteria are neither harmful nor helpful to us. However, quite a few are very necessary, such as the ones we call "nitrogen fixing bacteria". As you may know, air is made up of about 20% oxygen and 80% nitrogen.

All living entities need nitrogen for growth, but the nitrogen in the air is not suitable because it is in the form of gas which the plants cannot use. Nitrogen fixing bacteria convert the gaseous nitrogen in the air into an organic form of nitrogen which plants can use. Without these bacteria the soil would not be fertile and without fertile soil there would be no food.

Similarly, bacteria are used in the making of cheese and yogurt, in the production of beer and wines and for many other useful purposes.

As far as this handbook is concerned, we are going to concentrate on the harmful or pathogenic bacteria that cause food poisoning.

How do bacteria get on to our food?

We have seen that, for all practical purposes, bacteria are everywhere and that a minority of these are dangerous or pathogenic. Because we cannot see bacteria, we unfortunately cannot tell whether or not a particular item of food is contaminated with pathogenic bacteria by simply looking at it or smelling it.

It is worth examining briefly where pathogenic bacteria are most likely to be found. If we know where they are and how they get into the food chain, we can work towards preventing contamination where this is possible.

Many pathogenic bacteria are to be found in the intestines of humans, animals, and poultry. One of the reasons for this is because they thrive best at body temperatures. The food and water we have consumed since we were born is, for the most part, the source of the bacteria in our intestines. The kinds of bacteria we have in our intestines are dependent largely on the type of foods we eat. Animals and poultry similarly have bacteria in their intestines from the foods they eat.

So as to trace the route by which bacteria spread, let us take a number of examples of typical foods that we eat and examine how they might have become contaminated with pathogenic bacteria even before we purchase them:

Cattle on a farm may be fed with grain that has been contaminated by rats that have salmonella bacteria (salmonella is the most common type of food poisoning). After eating the contaminated grain, the cattle themselves may become infected with these pathogenic bacteria. If the cattle are then slaughtered there will be many opportunities during the slaughtering process when the salmonella can contaminate the meat that we will eat.

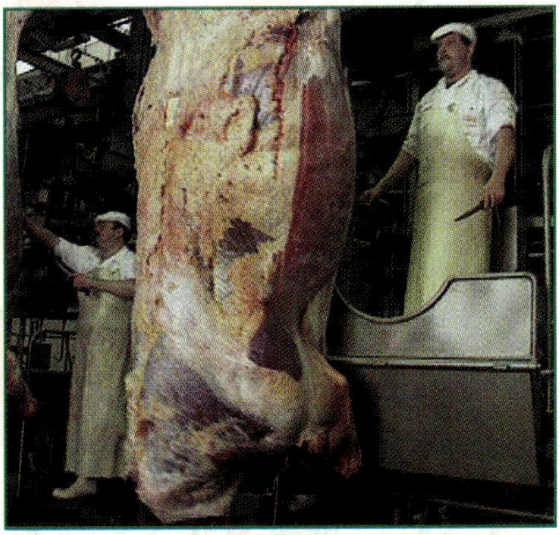

Unless food animals are hygienically handled after slaughter, the bacteria from their hides and intestines can directly contaminate the meat.

The hide of the animal is heavily contaminated with the salmonella from animal manure from the transport truck and the holding pens. If this hide touches the meat of the carcass, while the hide is being removed, then the meat will become infected. During the evisceration process, while the intestines are being removed, the intestines might be punctured or not properly tied off allowing salmonella organisms to escape and again contaminate the meat. Once the meat is contaminated then everything that comes in contact with it also becomes contaminated. This includes knives, work-tops, equipment or hands. And so, in this instance, salmonella contaminated beef arrives at a catering premises or butcher's shop or domestic kitchen. It will appear and smell the same as meat that is free of pathogenic bacteria. How it is subsequently handled, stored and cooked will determine whether it will go on to cause food poisoning.

Take **chicken** as another example: large numbers of chickens are slaughtered at the same time using the same equipment. If even one of these chickens is infected with pathogenic organisms then there is every likelihood that this chicken will contaminate the eviscerating machine. Once contaminated, the eviscerating machine will then go on to contaminate many of the remaining chickens in the batch.

Raw vegetables come from the soil. Some pathogenic bacteria occur naturally in the soil or they may be introduced into it by, for example, the spreading of animal slurry. This is why we should keep vegetables separate from other foods and take care to wash them thoroughly. In a food premises, they must be kept in a separate store, washed in a separate sink and prepared on their own work-tops, with equipment used only for vegetable preparation.

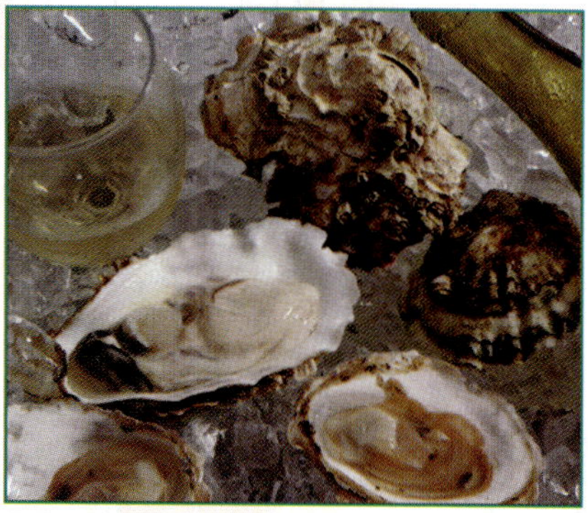

Shellfish such as mussels and oysters are considered high risk foods as they filter bacteria and viruses from the sea water.

Shellfish such as mussels, oysters, clams, scallops and cockles are called "bi-valve shellfish". The term "bi-valve" derives from the method by which these shellfish feed. They extract food from the sea water by filtering water through their flesh. They filter sea water in through one valve and after extracting nutrients and bacteria alike they expel the sea water through a second valve.

The flesh of the shellfish is, therefore, a filter that concentrates both pathogenic and harmless bacteria and viruses from the water. Naturally if the water in which they feed is even slightly polluted with sewage, or the like, then the flesh of the shellfish can be heavily infected. Some of these shellfish are eaten raw and therefore the living bacteria or viruses in their flesh go directly into our bodies.

Water is needed by all living entities. However, the water we drink passes through the ground and can pick up bacteria from the soil or from slurries, sewage or other pollutants. It can also pick up harmful chemicals which either occur naturally in the soil or are introduced by industry or farming.

Some of the greatest advances in public health protection and in the prevention of diseases have been brought about by the availability of clean, potable water. Today we often take this water for granted. However, we must always check that the water we use for drinking or food preparation is of a suitable health standard.

Most public supplies are disinfected to kill pathogenic bacteria and are safe to use for drinking, food preparation and cleaning provided they come directly from the rising mains and not through a roof tank.

However, many private supplies or private group schemes do not provide water that is suitable for use in a food premises unless it is further treated. If you are in doubt about the source or the quality of water to your premises then don't presume that it is satisfactory. Have it checked through the water analysing services provided by the Health Boards, the Local Authorities or an approved Laboratory. Remember too that, under the provisions of legislation governing the freedom of access to environmental information, you can request your Local Authority to send you copies of the analysis of samples that may have been taken from your supply.

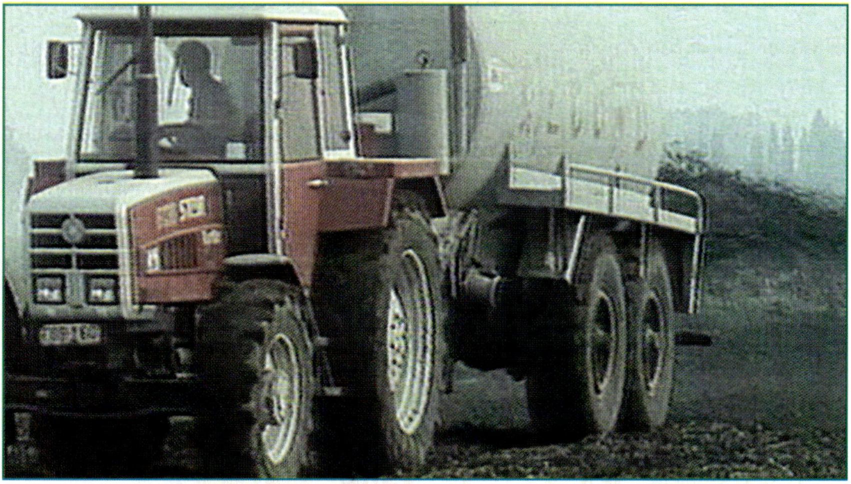

Water can be contaminated with animal or human slurries unless care is taken to ensure it is spread in a suitable location during good weather conditions.

At the time of printing of this book, up to 46% of private group water schemes in Ireland provide water that is in breach of European Union legislation on the quality of water for human consumption.

Milk is a highly nutritious food for pathogenic bacteria. In the past, raw milk from animals suffering from such conditions as tuberculosis sometimes resulted in people who consumed the milk also becoming infected. Thankfully the pasteurisation of milk has brought about a tremendous improvement in public health and in Ireland it is now illegal to sell cow's milk for direct human consumption unless it is pasteurised. Currently there is a trend to return to natural raw foods that are not processed in any manner. While such trends may have certain advantages from a nutritional viewpoint, it is important not to equate "raw" and "unprocessed" with "safe and wholesome". Milk is a case in point. Only pasteurised milk should be used for human consumption.

Intensively reared fowl have frequently been found to produce **eggs** which are already infected with pathogenic bacteria from the hen even before they are layed. Eggs should not be used for direct human consumption unless they have been suitably cooked or heat treated by, for example, hard boiling or pasteurisation.

How do bacteria grow?

The number of pathogenic bacteria a person consumes is one of the important factors that will influence whether the person gets food poisoning or not. If we know how bacteria grow, then by removing these suitable conditions, we can slow down or stop their growth or indeed by dealing with the food in a particular way we can provide conditions where the bacteria will be killed altogether.

Again, like all living creatures, bacteria need certain basic environmental conditions to enable them to grow and thrive. In particular these include the following:

- Suitable temperatures
- Moisture
- Food
- Time (to grow)

Temperature

Higher temperatures

Pathogenic bacteria grow best at our body temperature, i.e. 37°C. Bacteria multiply simply by one bacterium splitting into two bacteria. This process is known as binary fission. As mentioned previously this doubling in numbers can occur as often as every twenty minutes if there are

Cooking food so as to ensure all parts of it reach a temperature of 74°C, or above, for at least 2 minutes is a guaranteed way of killing bacteria such as Salmonella. All food workers preparing foods must remember this critical control temperature and time.

favourable conditions. If we increase the temperature above 37°C then the bacteria can still multiply but progressively more slowly. Their multiplication and growth can continue as far as 63°C. At this temperature (which is one that must be remembered by every foodworker) bacteria can no longer grow. Therefore, if you are keeping food hot it must be kept at or above 63°C.

If we raise the temperature as high as 74°C and maintain it for at least two minutes then we can actually kill off all bacteria. So if you are cooking food and want to be sure that any bacteria in the centre of the product are killed you must test the food to ensure that a centre temperature of 74°C is maintained for at least two minutes. In practical terms how can you check this?. Every food premises must have suitable probe food thermometers. The probe of the thermometer is pushed into the centre of the food and the temperature checked. If you don't use a probe thermometer you are only guessing - and guessing is not to be encouraged when it comes to food hygiene.

It can be seen, therefore, that a temperature of 74°C must be reached by all parts of the food for two minutes. This is sometimes difficult to achieve in large joints of meat or large catering-size turkeys, for example, because the outside can be overcooked while the inside may still not have reached anywhere near the temperature of 74°C. It is important that, where at all possible, portions of products such as meats should be kept to 2.5 Kgs maximum weight.

A most important principle of food hygiene, therefore, is that thorough cooking kills all living bacteria. This knowledge is an essential tool in preventing a premises from becoming involved in an incident of food poisoning.

However, it is important to remember that cooking will not make poor quality food into good quality food. While thorough cooking is an essential safeguard in preventing bacterial food poisoning, it is not a complete guarantee that the food is safe. There are two main reasons for this:

Some bacteria produce "spores" that are resistant to heat and these spores survive cooking.

Some bacteria produce a chemical waste product called a "toxin" that is also resistant to heat and cooking.

Spores

Certain types of bacteria produce spores. The best image I can use to describe what spores are is the image of an encapsulated bacterial seed that is protected in a hard shell. This shell protects the seed against conventional cooking and it is also resistant to many disinfecting chemicals. To illustrate the role of spores in food safety let us follow, say, a joint of meat that is contaminated with the bacteria that produce spores. We will take it that the food has been properly handled and stored before cooking so that the level of bacteria on the food is low. The meat is placed in a pre-heated oven for cooking. It is thoroughly cooked in that the centre temperature is maintained at 74˚C for two minutes- all the living bacterial cells are thereby killed. Now if the food is eaten directly after cooking then the food remains safe to eat. However if the food is, for example, required for a cold buffet the following day then how we deal with the food after it leaves the oven becomes critical. If the food is cooled rapidly and refrigerated then all is well. However if the food is left to cool in the warm environment of the kitchen then the spores that have survived the cooking germinate and grow into living cells. These bacterial cells will then go on to cause food poisoning if they are present in significant numbers. If you were to reheat the food again, it should be reheated so that it achieves a centre temperature of at least 70˚C.

Toxins

Toxins are chemical waste products produced by certain bacteria. These toxins are poisonous to humans. The toxins, like spores, are resistant to conventional cooking and therefore survive even in properly cooked food. People who consume food containing any significant level of toxins can often become violently ill very quickly after eating the contaminated food.

Low temperatures

We have seen how bacteria grow best at 37˚C and what happens to them as we increase the temperatures above this level. As we lower the temperature below this level bacterial growth progressively slows down. For food hygiene purposes we can take it that bacterial growth stops when we reach a temperature of 5˚C or lower. (Different textbooks will have slight variations on the baseline of 5˚C needed to stop bacteria from growing. While 5˚C is the most universally accepted temperature at which bacteria stop growing, the ideal temperature is between 0˚C and 3˚C. However for the purposes of this handbook we will consistently use 5˚C.) Thus it can be seen that bacteria grow between 5˚C and 63˚C. We refer to this range of temperatures i.e. between 5˚C and 63˚C, as the "Danger Zone". So as to minimise bacterial growth, therefore, food must be kept out of this "Danger Zone" range of temperatures as much as possible.

We use the principle of "Keep food hot (above 63˚C) or cold (below 5˚C) or don't keep it at all."

When bacteria are below 5˚C they don't grow but neither are they killed off at these temperatures and could instead be described as dormant. Refrigeration temperatures therefore must keep food below 5˚C.

Again the only way of knowing whether your refrigerators are maintaining food at this level is to check the temperature of the food using a suitable probe thermometer.

As we lower the temperature below 0˚C, food starts to freeze. Bacteria cannot grow when the temperature is below freezing. However, for the purposes of food hygiene, we can take it that freezing maintains bacteria in a dormant state but does not kill them. While bacteria do not grow when food is frozen, the food itself can still deteriorate in keeping quality unless it is kept at a temperature of below minus 18˚C. When foods are subsequently thawed and their temperature again increases above 5˚C, the previously dormant bacteria start to grow again.

This is why it is important to thaw foodstuffs in a fridge, unless they are defrosted on the defrost cycle in a microwave oven or are suitable for cooking directly from the freezer such as, for example, frozen chips.

Bacteria need food to grow

Like ourselves, all living things need food to grow and multiply. Bacteria grow best in nutritious foods because these foods are rich in protein, fats and carbohydrates and thereby provide the necessary building blocks for growth. Included in the grouping of nutritious foods are meats, dairy products, poultry, shellfish, soups, gravies, desserts, pastries and eggs. We should consider this group to be "vulnerable" foods as they are often involved in food poisoning outbreaks. Some types of bacteria have a preference for certain kinds of food.

Since our entire study in this handbook is on food hygiene and since our work involves food, we can take it that the elements required for bacterial growth are present all the time. Remember, too, that the "food" does not have to be present in large quantities - a spill of gravy on a worktop, as well as a drop of milk on a wipe cloth, is just as much a breeding ground for bacteria.

Moisture

All living creatures need moisture for growth. Where we remove moisture from food such as dried soups and custards, bacteria cannot multiply to any extent and the food will keep for much longer. However, as soon as we reconstitute the food by adding a liquid, then any bacteria in the food start to multiply again as if the moisture had never been removed in the first place. Foods which have a high salt or sugar content deny bacteria the moisture, which is more or less absorbed by the salt and the sugar.

Time

As we have seen, bacteria can double in numbers every 20 minutes or so under suitable conditions. Consequently, the more time that bacteria spend in such conditions, the greater the possibility that the food will subsequently cause food poisoning. As a rule of thumb, high risk foods that will not be cooked further before they are to be eaten should not be kept in the danger zone (between

5°C and 63°C) for more than one hour. Ideally these foods should not unnecessarily be in the danger zone at all.

Other factors influencing bacterial growth

There are some other factors that are outside of the scope of a handbook on the primary factors which influence growth of bacteria, such as the presence of oxygen, the presence or absence of preservatives, and the level of acid or alkali in a foodstuff.

Food spoilage

It is important to be able to distinguish "spoiled food" from dangerous or infected foods. We are all familiar with bananas turning black, bread going mouldy, various foods becoming rancid, and milk turning sour. These are obvious changes that we can see or smell and because of this we are not likely to eat them inadvertently. Consuming some of these foods such as black bananas or sour milk will probably not constitute a health risk but for the most part we will choose not to consume them.

Eating meat that has "gone off", on the other hand, would pose an unacceptable risk because of the vulnerability of the product and knowing that its condition may have been the result of bad handling or storage. This condition could also mean that pathogenic bacteria could have developed on the product to unacceptable levels.

Quite often the choice to eat some foods that are spoiled is a personal or indeed cultural choice.

Non-bacterial Contamination of Food

Viruses are incredibly small creatures, even smaller than bacteria, that can be consumed with food and cause illness. Viral forms of gastro-enteritis tend to develop rapidly after eating contaminated food and the symptoms often last no more than 24 hours. Even lower risk foods, such as lettuce, can be a source of viral infection. In such instances, because the surface of the lettuce is rough and usually wet and handled directly with our hands, we can literally wash off heavy loadings of viruses from our hands into the food. The study of viruses in any detail, though, is beyond the scope of this handbook.

Chemical contamination

Foods which contain certain chemicals or foreign objects can cause illness or injury when consumed. The chemicals may be introduced into the food at any stage of production, storage or preparation. At the growth stage, for example, meat can become contaminated with veterinary

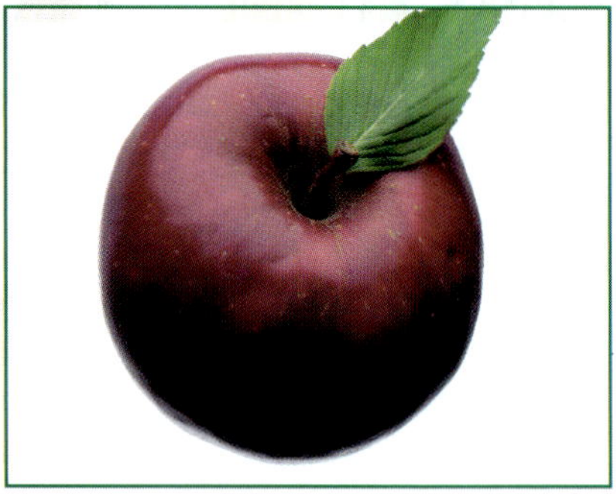

Pesticides and other chemicals can be present on the outside of fruits and vegetables. The foods should be properly washed before consumption.

drugs such as antibiotics or hormones. Crops can become contaminated with pesticides or fungicides. Most of these products can only be used provided a proper period of time is allowed to elapse between the application of the chemical and the slaughter or harvesting of the food respectively. The application of chemicals on fruit, for example, may be made on the presumption that the fruit will be washed before it is eaten. Chemicals may be added deliberately or accidentally. Such chemicals may be used in the wrong concentrations, at the incorrect time (too close to consumption) or on the understanding that the chemical will be washed off before eating. Any failure in this chain may result in the consumer becoming ill from chemical poisoning.

In recent years there have been many examples of chemicals being used deliberately to adulterate products, such as wine, so as to increase their weight or volume and some of these have resulted in widespread illness and poisoning.

In food premises, as well as in the home, it is essential that chemicals used for cleaning or other routine purposes are always kept in their original containers and never placed in containers used for the storage of foods. Great care must also be taken at all times to ensure that chemicals are not stored or used in such a manner as may permit their entry into food. The storage of certain acidic foods in copper or zinc-plated containers can result in these metals dissolving and contaminating the foods, causing subsequent poisoning. (We deal with chemical use in the food industry in more detail later.)

Accidental chemical poisoning is still very common. There are many cases in Ireland each year of chemicals being mistaken for foods, particularly by children. Also, some foods, such as mourel mushrooms and certain beans, contain natural poisons and these must be cooked in a certain manner to render them safe.

Physical contamination ... Foreign objects

The most common type of food complaint made to Environmental Health Departments relates to the finding of foreign objects in foods. These can vary from a loaf of bread containing a dead moth or rodent droppings to a piece of bacon containing a broken hypodermic or brine injecting needle. The subjects of these complaints occur through lack of care.

For example, a bakery with windows and doors that are not insect-proofed will inevitably have an insect in its products. A farmer who breaks the needle of a syringe when injecting a pig is blatantly putting consumers of the meat at risk if he does not have the needle removed by his veterinary surgeon.

(Taking precautions to prevent hazards that are associated with the food business is sometimes referred to as practising "due diligence" or may be dealt with under a system of hazard recognition and prevention known as "Hazard Analysis Critical Control Point" (HACCP). This will be dealt with in a summary manner later in the handbook).

Construction, maintenance or repair personnel working in a food premises frequently drop objects such as nails, pieces of wire, slivers of metal or glass, that fall either directly into food or into food containers. Such staff or visitors to your premises may not appreciate that their actions pose a threat to your business, so you must supervise their operations carefully. Remember that they are focused on their own work and are rarely trained in food hygiene.

Cross contamination

We have examined contamination of food by pathogenic bacteria, chemicals and physical or foreign objects. We have mentioned that while all of these are important the most significant is probably contamination with pathogenic bacteria. We have mentioned also that bacteria cannot move by themselves and rely on other means of transportation to get around.

To get on to food or to move from one food to another they use what we refer to as "vehicles" as a mode of transport. These vehicles can be such items as wipe cloths, work surfaces, cutting boards, knives and equipment, people, and other food. The transfer of pathogenic bacteria from one of these vehicles on to food is called cross contamination.

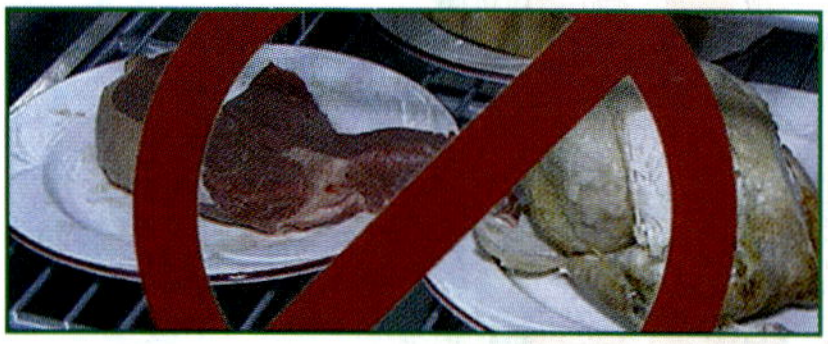

Cross contamination of food leads to bacteria from one food being transferred to another food. Particular danger arises if the food that becomes contaminated is "ready to eat" without further cooking.

Cross contamination can take place directly when, for example, raw meat touches cooked meat or a food worker sneezes directly on to food. It can also happen through what is referred to as drip contamination if, for example, raw meat is placed above cooked food in a refrigerator and blood containing bacteria from the raw meat drips down on to the cooked food thereby contaminating it.

Cross contamination can happen indirectly - for example, unwashed vegetables contaminating a work surface that in turn becomes the source of contamination on to the next food item placed on the same surface. Thus using different cutting boards for the preparation of the different categories of foods prevents cross contamination between these different foods. If the same cutting board must be used then it is essential that it is adequately washed and disinfected between uses. Similarly the use of separate equipment, wipe cloths and utensils for the different food categories is a means by which cross contamination can be prevented.

As already mentioned, people are the source of many food poisoning organisms. So if you don't wash your hands properly after using the toilet you can cross contaminate foods indirectly with bacteria from your intestine that have got on to your hands through soiled toilet paper.

If food premises are designed in a manner informed by a good knowledge of food hygiene, you will ensure that you provide zones for the storage and preparation of the different categories of foods and so minimise the risk of cross contamination.

(This is dealt with later in this book in the chapter on food premises design and layout on page 51).

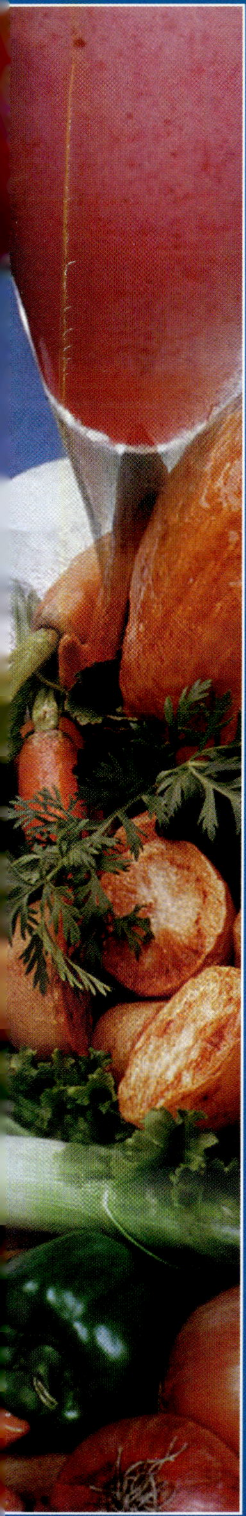

CHAPTER 3

FOOD POISONING

Food poisoning can be a serious illness especially in the very young, older people, those already ill and those who are pregnant. All food producers prepare food for these vulnerable groups of people.

Food Poisoning

As already mentioned, food poisoning is typically more than just an upset tummy that might be associated with overeating or indigestion. It is possible, though, that some people, having eaten fewer food poisoning bacteria or having a high immunity, may contract milder forms of the affliction and may not have any symptoms at all.

Typically, however, the sufferer is quite ill for anything from 24 hours to a few days or perhaps even weeks. Our immune system ensures that we can resist low numbers of dangerous bacteria fairly well but when we eat food with high levels of pathogenic bacteria or bacterial toxins then we will become ill. The most vulnerable to food poisoning are people who already have below normal immunity levels - these include:

1. Young Children
2. Older people
3. Those who are already ill, or who have some condition that has affected their immune response

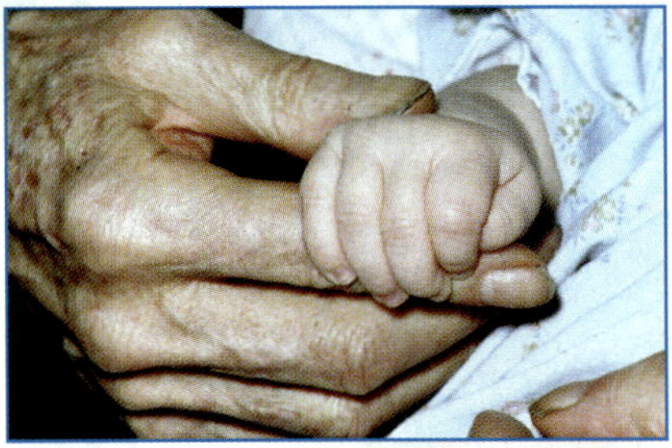

Young children and older people are most vulnerable and are at greater risk from food poisoning.

In addition pregnant women also have a vulnerability that can result in complications of the pregnancy.

While death from food poisoning in the developed countries is now fairly rare, when such deaths do occur it is more likely to be from the above groups. If you cater for any of these particularly susceptible groups, in a hospital or nursing home for example, then you must be even more particular than normal in taking food hygiene precautions.

However, almost all manufacturing, catering and retail premises provide foods for people from the susceptible groups, sometimes without being aware of it. For example, a person eating in your restaurant may look like a healthy adult but may actually have a medical condition that you are not aware of.

Kinds of Food Poisoning

There are three main types of food poisoning:

1. Infection
2. Intoxication or poisoning
3. Chemical poisoning

1. Infection

As its name suggests, this is where infection occurs within our gastro-intestinal tract. A good way to understand this is to recall what an infected cut looks like ... oozing and pus filled. The infection caused by food poisoning is exactly the same except that it is on the inside of the body. Consequently, people with infection type food poisoning often have pus or even blood in their diarrhoea. This type of food poisoning is also usually accompanied by a rise in body temperature.

The most common of all types of food poisoning, Salmonella, falls into this group. It takes some time for the infection to become established and it is usually at least 24 hours before a person becomes ill. The time between a person consuming the bacteria and showing symptoms of food poisoning is called the "incubation period".

2. Intoxication

Some bacteria, such as Staphylococcus aureus and Clostridium botulinum, do not cause an infection in themselves, but excrete a waste product, which is poisonous to consumers. Called toxins, these poisonous substances are not destroyed by conventional cooking. It is a commonly held misconception that thorough cooking of food always renders the food safe.

Thorough cooking is, of course, an essential food safety measure in relation to most forms of food poisoning, but not the intoxication type. Some forms of toxin type food poisoning, such as botulism, can cause death very rapidly. We can become ill very quickly after eating food containing these dangerous toxins, sometimes even before rising from the table after the meal.

3. Chemical poisons

Apart from the toxins produced by bacteria there are many other poisonous chemicals. If any such poisons are introduced to food then obviously the food becomes a vehicle for transporting the poison into our bodies. We have already looked at this type of poisoning in chapter 2 - Chemical Contamination.

Food-borne diseases

Apart from the above types of food poisoning, there are other conditions known as food-borne diseases. While bacteria responsible for infection or toxin-related poisoning actually grow in the food consumed, there are bacteria and viruses which may not grow in the food but use it as a means of entering our bodies, causing diseases and gastro-enteritis. Examples of these would include shigella and infectious hepatitis.

The most common causes that contribute towards food poisoning:

It is generally accepted that the following practices, in order of importance, contribute to the causes of food poisoning:

1. Food is prepared too far in advance of consumption and where it is subsequently stored improperly. The safest way to deal with food is to cook it thoroughly and serve it hot as soon after it is cooked as possible.
2. Cooling food too slowly. If food is cooked and then cooled too slowly, bacteria that either have survived improper cooking or bacteria that have contaminated the food after it is cooked will have the opportunity to grow as the food may be left in

the danger zone temperatures (between 5° and 63°C) for a longer than necessary period of time.

3. Not re-heating food to a high enough temperature. Food must be re-heated so that all parts of the food reach a temperature of at least 70°C.
4. The use of cooked food contaminated with food poisoning bacteria after cooking.
5. Under-cooking.
6. Inadequate thawing of food.
7. Cross contamination.
8. Storing hot food below 63°C.
9. Infected food handlers.
10. The use of leftovers.

The common types of Food Poisoning

It is not expected that food workers doing a primary course in food hygiene would know the signs and symptoms of the main types of food poisoning or how they may get on to our foods. It is important, however, that they would know a few of the names of the most common types and perhaps know a little more detail about a couple of them, such as Salmonella and E-coli H0157.

For reference purposes we will now deal very briefly with the more common types of food poisoning, and these include:

a) *Salmonella*
b) *E-coli H0157*
c) *Clostridium perfringens (also called clostridium welchii)*
d) *Clostridium botulinum*
e) *Staphlococcus aureus*
f) *Bacillus cereus*
g) *Listeriosis*
h) *Campylobacter*

In referring to preventative measures in the following paragraphs, all the food hygiene precautions mentioned separately in this handbook should always apply.

Salmonella

There are over 2,000 different types of Salmonella and each may vary somewhat in the severity of its symptoms.

Source

Salmonella food poisoning is predominantly associated with the consumption of infected poultry, meat, eggs, mayonnaise, mousse and dairy products. A significant percentage of poultry, pork and eggs is known to be infected with salmonella before arriving at food premises. This infection may also be picked up by poultry and other animals from infected feedstuffs, from other animals, especially in intensive rearing units, or even from rats or other rodents.

Salmonella can sometimes be transferred to food by a "carrier" ... somebody who is excreting the organism in the stools and who may or may not display symptoms.

Incubation period

As already mentioned, the incubation period is the time lapse between the consumption of the food containing the food poisoning organisms or toxins and the time at which a consumer shows the first symptoms. The incubation period for salmonella is normally between 12 and 72 hours but it can be as short as six hours and as long as one week.

Duration of the illness

It is not unusual for symptoms to persist for up to one week and sometimes even longer.

Symptoms

Symptoms include diarrhoea, vomiting, loss of appetite, a rise in body temperature and sometimes headache and aching limbs.

Prevention

Proper temperature control of food from the point of production through to the consumer's table.

Thorough cooking or heat treatment of foodstuffs, including pasteurisation of milk and liquid egg supplies.

Many animal feedstuffs should be suitably treated before consumption by animals. Swill, for example, must now be boiled.

Good animal husbandry on farms and particularly in intensive animal or poultry rearing units.

Good hygiene in slaughtering premises.

E-coli H 0157

This organism has only been identified and associated with serious illness within the past few years. Many of the members of the E-coli family are not harmful but a few are pathogenic to us. The dangerous members of the E-coli family produce toxins called verotoxins and these are extremely poisonous to humans. Up to 20% of people who contract E-coli H0157 develop a condition called HUS (Haemolytic Uritic Syndrome) which can cause serious damage to some of the major organs of the body, such as the kidneys.

A significant number of people - around 10% - can die from this condition, especially if they are in the vulnerable groups of people mentioned earlier. One of the other causes for concern about E-coli H0157 is that a very small number of the bacteria can actually cause somebody to become ill. It is thought that as few as five to ten bacteria may be sufficient to cause illness. This constitutes a miniscule dose when you consider that it may take thousands of Salmonella bacteria to cause illness. It is often thought that medical science has an understanding of how all these bacteria operate but the reality is that there is much about this particular bacteria that we don't understand at this time. Like many food poisoning organisms, the good news is that this bug can be killed by thorough cooking.

Source

While E-coli naturally occur in soil, the main source for the dangerous types is in animal slurries and in the intestines and on the hides of domestic food animals. These bacteria are easily transferred from contaminated animal hides or intestines on to the meat intended for human

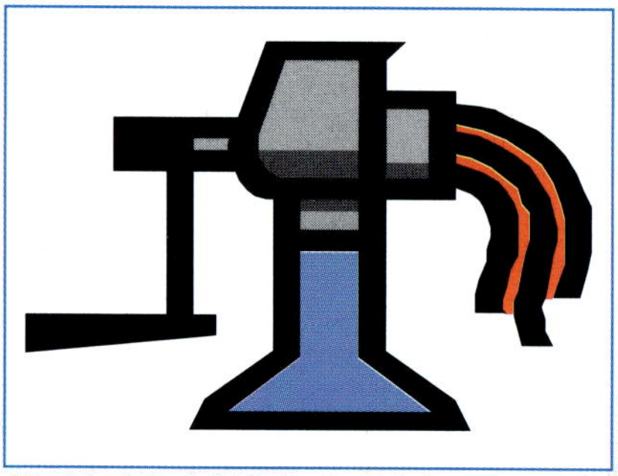

Mincing of meat distributes bacteria from the outside surfaces right throughout the batch. Minced meat, in any form, is particularly in need of thorough cooking.

consumption. Unless the meat or meat products are kept separate from foods intended for eating without further cooking, they can contaminate these high risk foods and cause food poisoning. Mincing or comminution of the meat enables the bacteria to be mixed right through all parts of the meat. Thus foods that are mainly made up of minced meat products such as burgers, minced meat itself and sausages are particularly high risk. If any of these products are handled directly or cross-contaminate other foods, directly or indirectly, then the other foods can obviously become contaminated and go on to cause this serious form of food poisoning. As mentioned, this is especially true if the foods contaminated are not going to be heat treated before consumption.

Incubation period

Can be from 3-8 days but usually 3-4 days.

Duration of the illness

Mild cases only last for a few days but in more severe cases patients can be ill for a number of weeks and of course long term serious consequences can occur for those who suffered from kidney failure.

Prevention

- Care must be taken to ensure that animals presented for slaughter should be as clean as possible. Suitable precautions must be taken during the slaughtering process to prevent the meat being contaminated from the hide, the intestinal contents or knives or equipment that may be contaminated during the processing of the carcass. The weasand and bung of slaughtered food animals must be tied off during slaughtering to prevent contamination of the meat.

- Products which are high risk foods, that is, ready to eat without cooking, should always be kept separate from raw foods so that cross contamination can be prevented. Preventing cross contamination in this way includes using separate equipment, utensils, and cutting boards for raw foods and cooked or ready to eat foods.

- Care must also be taken to ensure that food workers do not themselves cause cross contamination by handling raw foods and then ready to eat foods without first washing their hands properly. Preferably, there should be different food staff for these two separate categories of foodstuffs.

- Proper temperature control of vulnerable foodstuffs during all stages of storage and production.

- Thorough cooking of vulnerable foodstuffs.

- Fruit and vegetables should be properly washed before consumption.

Food workers must report to their supervisor any instances when they themselves suffer any form of gastro-enteritis or when people with whom they have significant contact, such as their family members, suffer from any gastro-enteritis conditions.

Clostridium perfringens

Source
This organism is widely found in soil and in the intestine contents of animals, humans and fish. This is one of the organisms which forms spores.

Incubation period
Very rapid with sudden onset of 6 - 24 hours.

Duration of the illness
Usually short with symptoms often abating after 24 hours.

Prevention
Normal good food hygiene practices such as serving food hot immediately after cooking. Proper general temperature control of foods. Using smaller joints or cuts of meat when cooking. Good personal hygiene.

Clostridium botulinum

Source
This spore-forming organism produces one of the deadliest toxins know to man. It can be found in the intestines of animals and humans.

Incubation period
May be from 12 hours to several days.

Duration of illness
Full recovery can take several months.

Symptoms
Blurred vision, often a sore throat, vomiting and diarrhoea. As the illness progresses paralysis can set in, particularly in the respiratory system. If left untreated the patient can die in up to 40% of cases. Death can sometimes be as a result of secondary infection.

Prevention
- Proper heat treatment and processing of foods in tins or jars and vacuum packed products.
- Blown or bulging cans should always be returned to the manufacturer unopened.
- Particular attention should be given to vacuum packaging of lightly salted or cured meats in non-processing premises in particular.
- Home preserving of foods should be discouraged unless the householder is aware of proper preserving techniques.

Staphylococcus aureus

Source
Normally found in a significantly high percentage of peoples' upper respiratory tract ... nose, mouth and throat. It is also found on our hands and especially in cuts, spots, boils and the like. The organism is introduced into the foods by sneezing, laughing, talking near open food and also from our hands after indulging in unhygienic habits such as nose picking, smoking, after handling a handkerchief or by failing to protect cuts and sores with

waterproof dressings. This is a toxin producing organism that can also be transferred through milk from cows with infected udders.

Incubation period
As with most toxin producers, the incubation period is short ... from half an hour to four hours but possibly up to 12 hours.

Duration of illness
24 - 48 hours.

Symptoms
Sudden onset, predominantly with vomiting and sometimes with diarrhoea. On occasions the body temperature is lower than normal.

Prevention
- Good personal hygiene.
- Good temperature control of food.
- Protecting foods from contamination by covering and protecting open food in public areas with sneeze barriers and the like.
- Exclusion of food handlers who may be a high infection risk due, for example, to severe acne or other skin infections.

Bacillus cereus

Source
This is a spore forming micro-organism, often associated with rice, which can be found naturally in soil and many foods.

Incubation period
From 1 - 12 hours.

Duration
Usually no longer than 24 hours.

Symptoms
There are two different types of toxins produced by this organism - one which is easily destroyed by heat and one which is not destroyed by heat. Symptoms of the former are predominantly diarrhoea, while the second usually causes vomiting.

Prevention
Proper temperature control of foods. For example, where a large batch of rice is prepared for later consumption, it should be cooled rapidly by rinsing in potable cold water and then refrigerated. It must then be reheated thoroughly before consumption.

Listeriosis

Source
The prevalence of the listeria organism and the acceptance of its significant role in causing food poisoning is relatively recent compared to other food poisoning organisms, with perhaps the exception of E-coli H0157. Much is still unknown about the organism and its exact mode of action. Listeria monocytogenes is the causative organism and could be considered both as a form of food poisoning and food-borne disease, as the organism can either grow on food or simply use food as a means of transportation.

Listeriosis can also be contracted without the involvement of food whatsoever, as it can be picked up directly from infected farm animals or their aborted foetuses or animal excreta. Listeria bacteria are also to be found commonly in soil, water and on vegetables. It is also believed that up to 5% of the population excretes the organism, even though they have no symptoms. And the organism can grow even in poor refrigeration, ie refrigeration above 5°C.

It is believed that the prevalence of the organism in food can be partly accounted for by the increase in the widespread storage of "convenience" or pre-cooked foods for longer periods under refrigerated conditions. The infection of farm animals with the organism is not uncommon and silage seems to be a significant reservoir for the infection.

People who suffer from acute listerosis are mainly those already mentioned in the risk groups earlier, ie the very young, older people, those already ill or on immunosuppressant drugs, such as steroids. However one of the most serious risk groups for this infection are pregnant women who can miscarry the foetus or have a stillbirth, and in some cases the newborn infant can suffer from the illness. Consequently there is a high risk of death.

Incubation period
The exact incubation period is unknown but it is thought to be between a few days and three weeks.

Duration of illness
Between 30% - 50% of those acutely infected can die. Recovery from the illness can be extremely slow.

Symptoms
Symptoms can vary from mild cases with flu-like symptoms to more serious cases with symptoms resembling those of meningitis, or perhaps septicaemia (blood poisoning). Infected lesions may also appear on the skin or in a number of sites within the body.

Prevention
Proper education of food handlers is required, particularly with regard to the need for correct temperature control of foodstuffs.

Adequate heat treatment of pasteurised or pre-cooked foods, with subsequent correct temperature storage of such foods. It is thought that pasteurisation temperatures should now be generally raised so as to be in excess of 76°C. Special care needs to be exercised in "cook-chill" or "cook freeze" food catering systems.

"Cook-chill" and "cook freeze" are terms used for the preparation of food by controlled pre-cooking of food, followed by rapid cooling and chilling, or freezing. Chilled food is kept for a maximum of five days at very low refrigeration temperatures and reheated immediately before use to a minimum temperature of 74°C for two minutes. The frozen food is thawed and reheated immediately before consumption to a minimum of 74°C for two minutes.

The Department of Health and Children has guidelines on these food preparation systems and anybody involved in this kind of catering will find the guidelines very worthwhile.

Pregnant women and immuno-compromised people should avoid contact with any potentially infected farm animals or their aborted foetuses, possibly contaminated silage or animal slurries. Access by very young children to farmyards and farm animals should be discouraged. Farmers and veterinary surgeons must exercise great care when working on farms and the precautions listed under " Common problems in the Home", in Chapter 10 should be borne in mind.

Pregnant women and immuno-compromised people should also avoid direct contact with anybody who is infected. They should also be discouraged from eating soft cheeses or pate, while minimising consumption of coleslaw and pre-cooked foods which have been stored in refrigerated conditions for extended periods.

Vegetables for human consumption should preferably not be fertilised with animal slurries. Very careful washing of vegetables is advised, together with the prevention of cross contamination of other foods with soil or vegetable material.

Further research still needs to be done to help us understand Listeriosis and its causes and prevention.

Campylobacter

This organism is also becoming increasingly identified as a source of food poisoning. It has been suggested that if all patients showing symptoms of food poisoning were thoroughly screened, then it is likely that this organism would show up as the most common source of infection ... even more common than we know Salmonella to be.

Source

Farm animals, household pets, rodents, birds and poultry, as well as unsuitably treated water and raw milk. Further sources include infected people, although this is rather unusual.

Incubation period

Usually 3-5 days but can range from 1 - 10 days.

Duration of illness

The majority of sufferers are over the acute symptoms in a few days but in one out of five cases illness may persist for a number of weeks and relapses can occur.

Symptoms

Diarrhoea, tummy cramps, nausea, vomiting and raised body temperature.

Prevention

- Good food hygiene precautions with proper food handling, thorough cooking and appropriate temperature control.

- Use only pasteurised milk and properly treated safe drinking water.

- Ensure that any domestic animals with an infection, especially diarrhoea, are treated promptly by a veterinary surgeon. Also ensure that infected pets are not handled, particularly by children. Routine thorough washing of hands after handling of raw poultry, pets or after contact with farm animals is essential.

Infected people must be excluded from food handling during acute illness.

General
There are many other organisms which can give food poisoning or food-borne disease but this handbook could not include them all. However, brief reference can be made to some of these.

Cryptosporidium
This is not actually a bacterium but it is a parasite called a protozoan. It is most commonly sourced from farm animals and pets, it can be transferred to humans either directly or through raw milk, water, food or from person to person. Young children, especially after another illness, are particularly vulnerable.

Giardiasis
Another protozoan that can spread from person to person, from animals or from contaminated water or food. It is important that any person with this condition visits their general practitioner to avail of specific treatment to eradicate the organism from the body.

Shigella (bacillary dysentery)
An extremely infectious condition that can rapidly spread from person to person, especially to children. Outbreaks can be explosive, even on an international basis. Significant portions of the population in an outbreak-affected area can be ill. Most cases are relatively mild but a small number can be prolonged and severe. Good personal hygiene, especially in nurseries, pre-schools, schools and institutions are the best means of control.

Examples of Food Poisoning Cases

I will briefly outline the events leading to two separate outbreaks of food poisoning. While you read the accounts of the events try to spot the poor practices that might have contributed to causing the outbreak. While the cases are based on fact, the names are fictitious.

Case 1.
Mr. and Mrs. Smith live with their three children, aged 7 years, 6 years and 18 months. Their normal Sunday dinner is centred around a roast chicken. The fresh chicken was purchased on a warm Saturday afternoon and was left in the boot of the car for two hours while Mrs. Smith completed the rest of the shopping. On arriving home the chicken was placed in the refrigerator along with a considerable quantity of other foods which were to supply the family for most of the following week. The refrigerator was found later to be achieving a temperature of 12°C in normal operation.

The chicken was transferred directly from the refrigerator to the oven around 11.30 am on Sunday morning and the oven switched on. By 1.00 pm the chicken appeared to be cooked and was served directly. All except the 6 year old ate some of the chicken at that meal. All the chicken was not eaten and the left-overs were put back into the "switched off" oven until the family returned from their Sunday outings at 7.00 pm at which time Mrs. Smith and the 18 month old child ate what was left of the chicken directly from the "cold" oven.

At 1.00 pm the following day the 18 month old child did not eat his dinner and was subsequently very ill from around 3 pm for five days with diarrhoea and a raised temperature. During this time the family doctor sent a stool specimen to the local laboratory who later confirmed salmonella food poisoning.

Mrs. Smith became ill herself two days after eating the chicken but had a relatively mild version of the illness compared with the child and had seemingly recovered in 48 hours. The rest of the family did not become ill - they were lucky that time. The recovered chicken carcass of the cooked chicken was found to contain the same Salmonella bacteria as had been isolated from the child.

The usual plea that the family had often treated the Sunday chicken in this way in the past without causing a problem was little consolation to the very ill child - the innocent victim of lack of knowledge or failure to put that knowledge into practice.

How many food hygiene mistakes were made in dealing with this chicken after the time of purchase?.

Case 2

A busy hotel was having a good summer season and not only were all its rooms occupied but it also had a wedding reception. Because the kitchen was under a lot of pressure, it had to start cooking the large catering sized frozen turkeys on Monday for the wedding reception on the following Wednesday. Two turkeys were thawed in the kitchen sink overnight on Sunday. The next morning the partly thawed birds had to be removed from the sinks and placed on a tray in the dry goods store.

The ovens were in constant use during the day and the two turkeys were cooked immediately after lunch on Monday. After cooking they were left in the kitchen overnight to cool and put into the cold room on Tuesday morning. Subsequent to these turkeys, various other sets of turkeys were cooked. They were removed from the cold room at 1 pm on the following Wednesday, sliced, apportioned and placed on serving trays. The reception was to commence around 2.30 pm and the chef, knowing how unpredictable weddings can be, awaited the arrival of the wedding party at 3.45pm before placing eight large apportioned turkeys into the ovens for reheating, together with a large quantity of cooked ham.

Of over 200 guests, about 40 were ill within 24 hours. Almost all the "top table" were affected, including the newly-married couple - not the most pleasant way to spend a honeymoon. Clostridium perfringenes was isolated from the affected patients who were tested and also from the carcasses of two of the turkeys.

What were the incorrect procedures which contributed to this outbreak?.

Step by step, could you say what should have been done?.

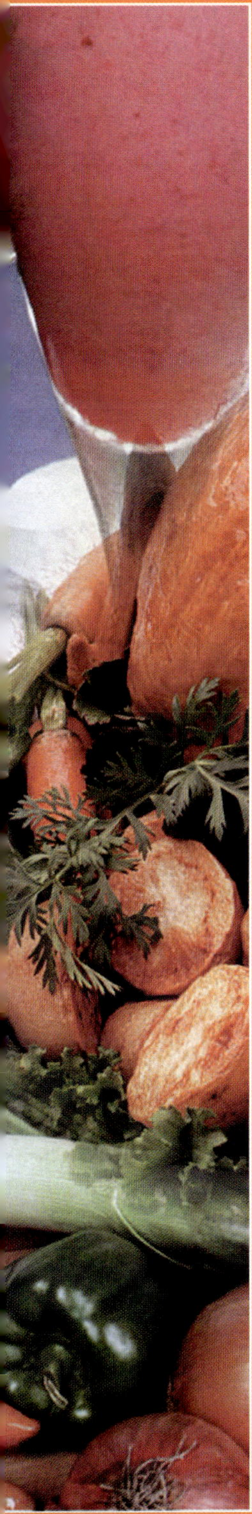

CHAPTER 4

FOOD PURCHASE, DELIVERY, STORAGE AND PREPARATION

Purchasing foods from reliable suppliers who deliver good quality food in hygienic transportation is an essential starting point to producing or selling safe food from your own premises. Storing food properly after delivery prevents bacteria from growing.

Food purchase, delivery and storage

Now that we know why food hygiene is important and have some idea about pathogenic bacteria and food poisoning, let us examine in some detail other important hygiene considerations when dealing with food, from delivery through to consumption. Bear in mind that this handbook is not exhaustive and deals only with the basic practices and common problems regularly encountered by Environmental Health staff when they are inspecting food premises.

Purchase of food

It is essential that food products are purchased only from reliable suppliers who can be depended on to supply wholesome, safe food. New suppliers, with "unbeatable bargains" of vulnerable foodstuffs should, as a matter of course, be treated with suspicion. Unscrupulous suppliers might try to sell you foods which others have rejected as inferior or products that are dangerous.

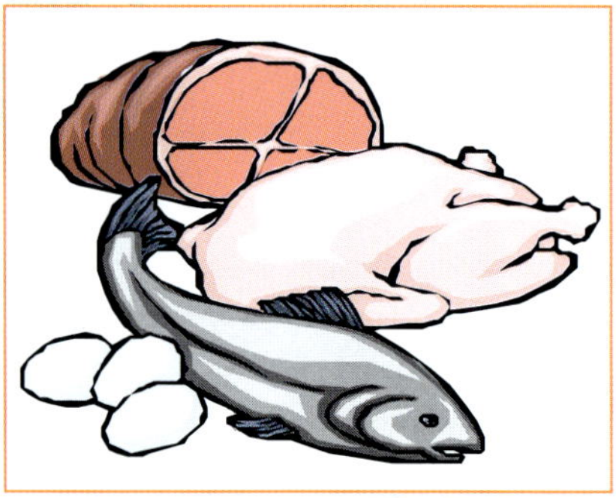

The quality and safety of food you sell from your premises is dependent on the quality and safety of food you purchase.

Your business and reputation is dependent upon the quality and safety of the food that you sell. Thus the quality and safety of the food that you purchase should be a primary consideration for you. Remember that no matter how well you look after food hygiene safety measures in your own premises, you are dependent on the measures already taken in your suppliers' premises - you cannot transform poor quality or unsafe food into high quality safe food.

Where possible you should consider purchasing foods only from premises that you inspect yourself or which you have had independently audited for you, if you are one of the larger premises with such resources. This is one way of being as duly diligent as you can be. If you do inspect suppliers' premises, ask them to outline to you the main risks associated with the types of foods that you are purchasing from them and then ask them to show you how these risks are either eliminated or minimised. You should feel free also to ask them to show you their quality control programme and, if they have any samples of their foods tested, ask to see the results. If you are not sure how to interpret the laboratory results, put the onus on the supplier to have the appropriate laboratory indicate to you the standards that the foods should attain.

You will not be in a position to do this for all your suppliers but do consider it for vulnerable foods, especially cooked meats and other ready to eat foods that are high risk.

Planning your purchasing

When you are choosing your supplier, one of the factors to bear in mind is whether they can supply you at a time that suits you. This is essential so that staff are available at your premises to inspect the goods as they are delivered and so that they can be brought directly into the appropriate store area.

Deliveries of foodstuffs should always be well planned so that sufficient space is available to accommodate them. This is very dependent, of course, on the style of management and your proximity to the markets. There is no point in buying in a week's or a month's supply of particular products that can be delivered at the same cost every other day. It is wasteful to keep a coldroom of 8 cubic metres working constantly when a room half the size would be sufficient with more frequent purchasing. It would also reduce cleaning demands.

Peak demands often arise at holiday weekends when extra capacity may be needed, but in these instances it would be better and cheaper to have a second refrigerator to be put into service only on these occasions.

Similarly, for example, there is little point in buying large quantities of frozen products such as poultry which can occupy valuable kitchen, freezer and thawing space if fresh products are available each day at or close to the same price.

Supply specifications

Many larger retail stores, catering establishments, hospitals etc. have food specifications as part of their contracts with suppliers. Supply specifications may include: the quality of the food (perhaps its ingredients), and conditions under which it is supplied (such as temperature control). It can sometimes include a warranty that accepts responsibility for any defects in the food over which the retailer or caterer has no control but for which they can be subsequently liable to their customers.

Such specifications are to be recommended and more establishments should implement them as a purchasing requirement. They need not be too detailed as even simple specifications can prove most beneficial. For example, if you were purchasing fresh lamb carcasses from a wholesale supplier, you could include something such as the following conditions in your purchase agreement:

- "No lamb over (specify age) shall be supplied under the description of lamb.
- The lamb shall be hygienically slaughtered in a licensed abattoir under veterinary supervision.
- All lambs shall be veterinary inspected before and after slaughter and must bear the "health mark" stamp on the carcass.
- All lamb shall be stored in refrigerated conditions under 5°C for a maximum of (specify period) of days prior to delivery.

- Lamb carcasses shall be hung from hooks during transportation and not stored on the floor of any vehicle.
- Lamb carcasses shall be delivered to (specify premises) on the following days ....between the following times.....
- Staff at the abattoir and those involved in delivery shall be suitably trained in the hygienic handling of the meat and shall always be suitably attired in clean outer clothing while engaged in the food business.

  Such staff shall at no stage engage in any unhygienic practice while working with the food or in my food premises.
- The supplier shall hereby warrant that the lamb as supplied does not contain any substances that are unacceptable to the consumer or that might render the food to be unfit or unsafe or of less than the highest standard.
- Meat as supplied shall be kept in refrigerated transport vehicles only and the vehicles shall ensure that the meat is delivered at a temperature of less than five ° Centigrade.

  Product delivered at a temperature above this limit shall be rejected at the loss of the supplier.
- The transport vehicle shall be used solely for the conveyance of food and shall be kept clean and in good repair at all times.
- The lamb carcasses shall be weighed and inspected individually by a nominated person in my premises at the time of delivery".

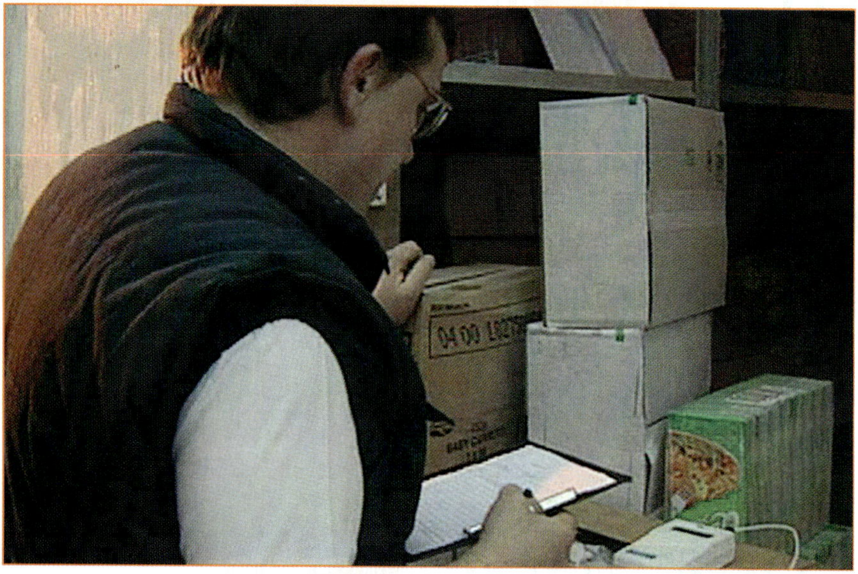

Reject any deliveries of vulnerable foods that are not delivered at appropriate temperatures.

Recording deliveries

It is essential that you are able to trace any foodstuffs that are delivered to your premises. This is especially important where foods are withdrawn from sale because they were found to be dangerous or from premises that were found to be a high risk of serious food contamination. You are legally obliged to identify suppliers of food to your premises and indeed the sources to which you supply also, with the exception of retail sale, of course.

Delivery vehicles

These should be checked as a matter of routine to ensure that the food you are purchasing from the vehicles is protected and weather proof during transit. Check that the vehicle is in good repair, especially the doors opening into the food storage compartment. Remember that faulty doors can result in dirt, carbon deposits and exhaust fumes being vacuumed into the vehicle and on to the food or food packaging. Check that the vehicle is pest proof, clean, has easily cleanable surfaces and shelving and does not have any non-food items stored in the food compartment, especially items that might contaminate or taint the food.

Ensure that the spare wheel is not stored in a position where it might contaminate food. Verify that the driver's cab is separate to the food compartment and that as a general rule no food is stored on the floor of the vehicle, especially unwrapped food. And, of course, ensure vehicles used for transporting refrigerated or frozen foods are designed for this purpose and that the food is at the appropriate temperature. Ensure that raw and cooked foods or ready to eat foods are stored in such a manner as will guarantee that there is no danger of cross contamination between the different categories of foodstuffs.

Inspection of deliveries

Your premises must have a system whereby there is a nominated person(s) to inspect food during the course of its delivery to your premises. Food must be visually inspected to check that its condition is satisfactory. As mentioned the delivery vehicle and the attire of the personnel making the delivery should be checked also.

Frozen foods should be checked to ensure that they are still hard frozen and are at or below a temperature of minus 18°C. Any foods that are in the process of thawing should be considered for rejection. Ensure that frozen foods are marked as "frozen" as occasionally product that was originally intended for sale as "fresh" and was not sold quickly may be frozen to extend its shelf life. When this food is subsequently thawed it may well be on the verge of "going off".

Refrigerated foods should preferably be delivered below 5°C. Check the colour and, if appropriate, the odour. Ensure that there is an appropriate span of time left before the "use by" date that indicates the end of the product's shelf life. Every premises should have adequate numbers of calibrated probe thermometers to check the delivery temperature of foods.

Canned foods should be free of dents or rust, since this kind of damage could allow air to enter the container, leading to conditions which could cause food poisoning. Cans that are "blown" (swollen beyond their normal size) should not be used and should be returned to the manufacturer unopened. Cans that are improperly labelled or have no labels at all should be rejected.

The labels of **dried foods** should be checked and boxes and packaging visually inspected to verify that they are free of any evidence of damage from rodents and from infestation by insects. Burst or leaking packages or containers should not be accepted into your premises. It is good practice to decant most types of food supplied in bulk: this means transferring it from original containers to fresh ones. Some containers may have become soiled in transit or from seepage of liquid from the contents.

In such cases, the undamaged contents should be transferred to washable boxes or trays at the time of delivery. Apart from providing an opportunity to inspect the food more carefully, this practice ensures that pests are discovered immediately and that premises are not contaminated by dirty packaging. Please ensure, however, that if you are decanting product that you preserve any details on the boxes or containers that are not replicated on the individual food item's packaging. This ensures that you can trace the origin, batch number or production code if necessary at a later stage.

For manufacturing businesses, it is necessary, for quality control purposes, to have samples of the food ingredients supplied to your business tested by a suitable laboratory on a regular basis. You must be satisfied that these tests are carried out independently on behalf of your suppliers and that the test results are available to you.

Food labelling

If food is delivered in packs or containers and sold to customers in those same packages then certain basic details should appear on the food label printed on the packaging. It is important to remember, however, that there are some exceptions to these details for certain products and remember that "wholesale" sale has somewhat different rules to "retail" sale: some of the details, for example, can be on the trade invoices. The illustration of a food item, such as a wrapped loaf of bread produced for retail sale, may best show the details normally required on the label or wrapper:

1. The name of the food ... "white sliced loaf".
2. A list of ingredients in descending order of weight - in this case one would expect to find "wheat flour" as the first ingredient.
3. A date of minimum durability, such as shown under the description of "use by".
4. The net weight of the product - such as 800 grams.
5. The name and address of the manufacturer or supplier or wholesaler or retailer.
6. Any special storage conditions.

Other requirements in some cases may be the country of origin, special preparation instructions and so on. As mentioned, this is only a rough guide and is only intended for use as such. A full study of the Labelling Regulations is needed if you are responsible for designing labels for foods.

Food storage

All deliveries should be made at a time when they can be brought to the appropriate store within the premises without any undue delay. In addition to the precautions mentioned above there are a number of principles that should be borne in mind for all food storage and these include:

Stock rotation

New stock should normally be stored in such a manner as will facilitate the use of the older stock first - first in - first out. This could mean placing new deliveries to the back of shelves or at the base of a chest freezer so that the older stock is more available to be used first. However, stock rotation must take account of the "best before" or "use by" dates on the packaging so that the older stock is used first even if it is delivered last. Where you are wrapping foods in the premises for storage purposes, such as storing food in a freezer, you must indicate on the wrapping the identity of the food and the date it was first stored. Stock must be regularly checked to ensure that any short dated stock is used quickly or that out of date stock is removed and disposed of.

There are a number of separate food stores within food premises.

These include:

1. Dry goods store
2. Refrigerated store
3. Freezer store
4. Fruit and vegetable store

Dry Goods Store

The potential hazards that might arise in dry goods storages areas include: possible bacterial growth due to cross contamination or excessive moisture, and contamination by pests or chemicals. It has already been stated that all foods should be closely examined on delivery and unsatisfactory goods or presentation rejected. The dry goods store holds foods such as flour, sugar, tinned foods, seasoning and so on. It is important to remember that it is a food store and should be used for food only. The room should be bright, well ventilated and reasonably heated in damp or cold weather. Shelving should be easy to clean and preferably on castors to facilitate cleaning. Good quality shelving, such as stainless steel, is more expensive in the short term but can work out cheaper in the end.

Dry goods should be stored well off the ground with the heaviest items on the lower shelves. Goods should not be left leaning against an outside wall. Like all other parts of the catering area, windows should have efficient insect screens.

Opened packages of food such as flour or sugar should always be stored in well-sealed bins. This helps to keep them dry and safe from insects and rodents. Bin storage also prevents spillages on shelving.

Cleaning materials should never be kept in a food storage area as there is a risk of contamination of foodstuffs.

Refrigerated Storage

The potential hazards that arise because of lack of suitable refrigeration or poor storage within refrigerators include: possible bacterial growth if suitable temperatures are not maintained and cross contamination between foods. Adequate space must always be available for all foods needing refrigeration. If space is limited there is a risk of cross-contamination with other foods or some food will, inevitably, be left out of the refrigerator altogether. Appropriate use of refrigerators or cold rooms can exercise a "critical control" of vulnerable foods and prevent bacterial growth during food storage.

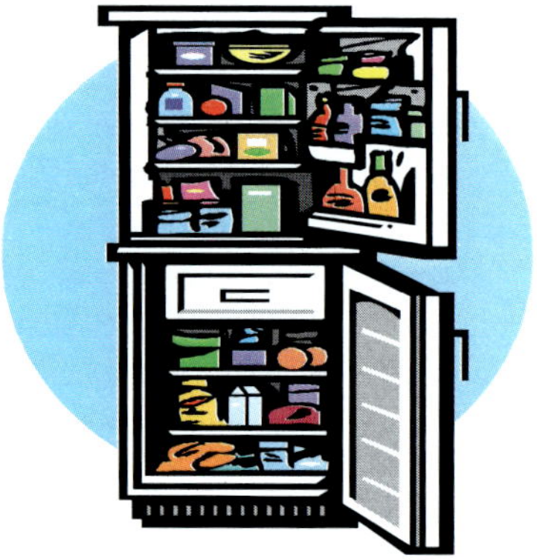

It is essential that refrigerators and freezers are not overstocked so that cross-contamination is less likely and that air circulation can take place.

Any refrigerator or cold room is only as good as the temperature it maintains and refrigerated storage can generate a false sense of security if proper temperatures are not achieved .

So how do you know if your refrigerator is working properly? Obviously, it should have a display thermometer which shows at a glance that it is operating between 0°C and 5°C. As already mentioned, all food establishments should also have a suitable number of calibrated probe thermometers to check the temperature of the food itself.

Within the coldroom/refrigerator all foods must be segregated so that:

1. Cream products, desserts, pastries etc. are stored on the uppermost shelves.
2. Cooked foods are stored immediately beneath the above items.
3. The next available shelves contain raw meats.
4. Washed fruit and salad vegetables are stored on the lowermost shelves.

Carcass meat or joints hanging in a cold room should not overhang other produce which could be contaminated by blood drips and they should not be hung where they could be contaminated by people entering the cold room. It is worth placing trays on the floor beneath carcass meat to allow regular removal of blood drips without having to continually clean the floor. In larger premises, of course, it makes more sense to provide separate cold rooms or refrigerators for different categories of food, such as raw meats and cooked meats. Many establishments also keep a separate refrigerator for fish to avoid tainting other foods.

Hot foods should never be stored in the refrigerator as this raises the temperature of the unit, and other food, and can cause condensation resulting in cross contamination between foods.

Too many establishments store vegetables and fruit unnecessarily under refrigerated conditions. Of course, refrigeration adds to the shelf life of some of these products by slowing down enzyme activity.

However, as previously mentioned, where regular deliveries are available valuable refrigeration space should not unnecessarily be used for vegetable products. Also bear in mind that many vegetables are heavily contaminated with soil and their packaging may also be contaminated, thereby posing a real risk to other vulnerable foodstuffs within the refrigerated facility. Ideally only washed fruit and vegetables should be stored in a refrigerator or cold room unless it is maintained exclusively for such purpose. Self-closing devices should be fitted on cold-room doors and many modern cold-rooms also have an indicator to show when the defrost cycle is operative.

Modern cold rooms have durable metal-clad, joint-free, washable walls, as well as joint-free, hygienic and easily cleaned floors and ceilings. All shelving should be of suitably coated metal and easily removed for cleaning. Thankfully, the number of cold rooms with wooden or concrete walls is rapidly decreasing and I believe there is no place for these in hygienic premises. Motor condensate from cold-rooms should be piped to an outside waste outlet, rather than collected in a bucket or basin which has to be regularly emptied and is sometimes forgotten, resulting in flooded floors.

Cold-room motors should always be provided with proper ventilation to remove generated heat - otherwise motor life is reduced and electricity costs increased. It is preferable that cold-room motors are sited externally to the premises or otherwise the motor ventilation grills must be insect and rodent proofed. Systems which use heat from cold-room motors to produce hot water, in larger premises, are to be encouraged and can pay for themselves within a year. However, bear in mind that if such a system is installed it must be supplemented, particularly during cold weather when the motors are less active and, therefore, unable to provide water at the necessary temperature for wash-up sinks and the like.

Many open, dairy-type refrigerated display cabinets achieve poor temperatures, with wide variations from shelf to shelf. Again, a probe thermometer is the only sure way to spot the variation. Many such cabinets are incorrectly positioned within retail areas and are affected by cross draughts and warm lighting, as well as by over-stocking which prevents proper air circulation. Suitable insulating plastic curtains are now deservedly growing in popularity for refrigerated self service display cabinets.

Deep-Freeze Storage

When placing unfrozen foodstuffs into a deep-freeze unit, care must be taken to ensure that the temperature of the freezer is not adversely affected. Therefore, only small quantities should be put in at any one time. Larger premises may have a separate unit, such as a blast freezer, for freezing food only. Deep-freeze rooms similar in structure to the modern cold-room are now also very popular and indeed hygienic.

All food placed in deep-freeze units should be properly sealed in order to:

a) prevent it contaminating or being contaminated by other foods, and

b) to prevent it drying out or being freezer burnt.

Foodstuffs in deep-freezers should always be properly labelled. Chest-type deep-freeze units pose a number of particular problems. Stock rotation is difficult because many items find their way to the bottom of the unit and may never be seen again! If the freezer is greater than 0.8m cubed in capacity, or the freezing area is over about 0.8m. in depth, it becomes tiresome to remove all existing stock in order to place new stock on the bottom of the unit. Many such units are under utilised with the upper half of the food stock being rotated and the bottom half forgotten.

Obviously, upright units which show the food stored at a glance are much more desirable and easier to manage, as are deep-freeze rooms. All chest-type deep-freeze cabinets should be sited at least 225mm off the ground to allow for air circulation and should also be movable for easy cleaning.

Similarly, food stored in freezers should be arranged to allow for air circulation. Because even sealed packets of foodstuffs become torn in freezers when knocked hard against other packets, it is important to separate different categories of food, either within the units or by using separate freezer units for each type of food if there are large storage requirements.

One of the most common faults found with freezers is that the air seal is lost because the gasket around the lid or door is damaged or worn. This results in freezers frosting up too quickly, wasting electricity and failing to maintain appropriate temperatures. These gaskets should be checked regularly and renewed when necessary. It is important to place thermal covers over open-top freezers during the night.

Another common problem relates to overstocking of open chest-freezers in retail sales areas, often causing load-lines to be ignored. Particular products lend themselves to this problem, such as frozen turkeys. Turkeys have a shape that makes them difficult to accommodate and even though they can be packed well by the retailer, customers soon disturb the orderly pattern and many birds are left above the load line. These in turn partly thaw and are refrozen again and again, posing a real risk to customers.

The obvious answer is to reduce the number of turkeys in the units, selecting a representative display of the range available and replenishing frequently as stock is purchased. It is not acceptable to allow mechandisers from suppliers to fill your deep freeze units above the load lines - the ultimate responsibility rests with you in your own premises, so keep a close check on suppliers when they are stocking these units.

Freezers must be maintained at a temperature of minus 18°C or below.

There is one exception to this for ice cream that is being kept in the premises for retail sale. In such instances a temperature of minus 12°C or lower is accepted.

Remember that foods which have been thawed may not be refrozen unless they have been cooked after defrosting.

Fruit and Vegetable Store

Fresh vegetables pose a special problem in catering and retail establishments due to the large quantities of soil which they or their containers may carry into the premises. Other hazards associated with fruit and vegetable stores includes the potential for spoilage caused by damp or humid conditions. Many businesses purchase only vegetables which have been substantially washed and this, of course, is to be advocated. Washed fruit and vegetables should be stored separately and may need to be re-washed before use in case they have become contaminated with dusts etc. from other items in the store.

All fruit and vegetables, with the possible exception of certain washed salad items needing refrigeration, should be kept in their own store, separate from all other foods. As with the dry goods store, this area should be well lit and vented. Sacks and other containers should be stacked on washable shelving or plastic pallets which allow for easy cleaning beneath and around the stock and to allow for good air circulation. It is preferable to have a vegetable store which has a separate area that can also be used for vegetable preparation, with washing sinks and good quality work-tops. Suitable traps and sedimentation chambers should be fitted to the drainage system serving vegetable preparation sinks to prevent vegetable particles and starches clogging drains. Many premises have out-buildings for storing vegetables but these are often below required standards. Like all food stores, vegetable stores must be insect and rodent proofed.

In retail establishments, vegetable sales areas should be substantially separate from sales areas for vulnerable foods. All too often packets of lettuce are seen in the refrigerated meat display unit, as indeed are boxes of mushrooms.

Cleaning Stores

A separate room should be provided for stocks of cleaning materials. As already mentioned, chemicals and foods should never be stored together because chemicals may contaminate or be mistaken for food.

Under no circumstances should chemicals ever be stored in food containers, even if the containers are re-labelled. Labels can fall off. Chemicals must always be kept in their original containers and if they must be transferred to other vessels for dilution purposes then those vessels should be easily distinguishable from any food container and bear clear, permanent

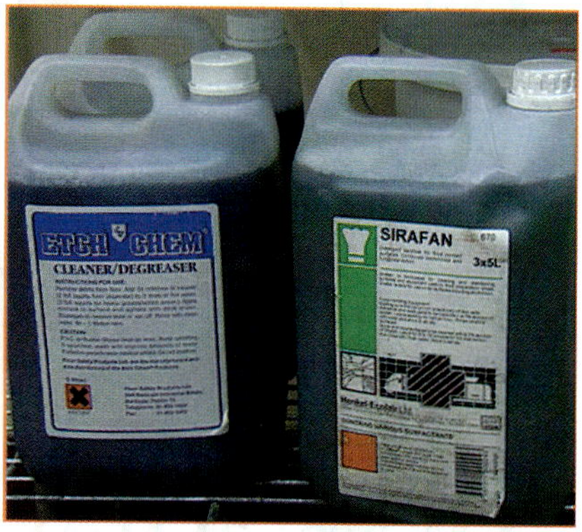

markings. Instructions for the use of chemicals and cleaning agents should always be available to cleaning staff, including such information as:

1. The purposes for which the product is suitable.
2. Its dilution factors.
3. Suitable methods of application.
4. Precautions to be taken when handling the product.
5. First aid precautions in case of an accident with the product.

A good cleaning store should have good lighting and ventilation, good quality, cleanable and sturdy shelving (especially at low levels for heavy containers) and a proper mop sink with hot and cold water. This store should always be kept secure. First aid equipment, such as eye washes, should be available in the first aid cabinet. Drums of chemicals which are fitted with dispensers are preferable to those which entail tipping over a 25-litre drum to pour caustic chemical into a cleaning bucket, with the associated risk of injury.

A proper mop sink ensures wash-up sinks are not used for mops.

Naturally, proper protective clothing for staff, including footwear, aprons, gloves and goggles, where necessary, should be readily available.

Food preparation, cooking and service;

We have now examined how food should be purchased and stored and so we move on to examining how we can minimise the risks to food during preparation, cooking and service. Again taking the example of catering premises serves to illustrate the safety principles in a manner that can be applied to any food preparation.

The main areas of concern, apart from those already covered, are: Defrosting of frozen foods, prevention of contamination of food during preparation, serving and holding food after cooking, cooling and freezing food, and using a microwave oven.

Defrosting of food

Small items of food such as frozen chips, vegetables etc. are often intended for cooking directly from the freezer. In this instance it is essential that the manufacturers instructions are followed closely. Allowance must be made for the additional time that it takes to cook from frozen as distinct from fresh. This method is obviously not suited to the cooking of larger food items.

Most foods coming from the freezer must be defrosted/thawed in a refrigerator. The reason for this is simply that the outside of the food defrosts first while the inside is still frozen. This means that bacteria on the outside can start to multiply rapidly unless the food is stored outside of the danger zone i.e. in the refrigerator. Defrosting frozen foods, such as meat, in water gives a similar concern in relation to presenting bacteria with an environment where they can easily grow. If food is defrosted in water not only can the food become contaminated with the water but the exudate from the defrosted food will also contaminate whatever container is used, such as a kitchen sink. The resultant potential cross contamination risks are inherently dangerous.

Defrosting may also be carried out in a microwave oven that has a defrosting cycle. It is essential that the manufacturers instructions are followed in this case as microwave ovens vary considerably in power output and the time needed to defrost different food items. As with any form of defrosting, apart from those intended for cooking directly from the frozen state, it is necessary to ensure that the food is totally defrosted before cooking is commenced. The only way to do this effectively is to use a probe thermometer to ensure that the centre of the food is at a temperature above freezing. If improperly defrosted food is cooked then some of the heat that should be used for cooking will actually be used for defrosting allowing bacteria not only to survive in the centre but possibly even multiply.

Once food is defrosted it is should not be refrozen again unless it is first cooked.

Preventing contamination during preparation.

As will be referred to in more detail in chapter 5, it is necessary to prepare different categories of foods on different worksurfaces while using different utensils so as to prevent cross contamination. During active preparation, foods will generally be in the main kitchen environment and the temperature of this environment will be in the danger zone. It is essential that food is not left in this temperature for too long, so large quantities of foods should not be taken out of the refrigerator at any one time. It is safer to take out only smaller quantities that can be prepared quickly before taking more food into the danger zone environment. When food is cooked it should either be served or kept hot (above 63°C) or alternately cooled quickly and refrigerated.

Work-surfaces should be sanitised before food comes in direct contact with them. Any foods that need to be washed must be washed in potable water only. After washing such items as cabbages and lettuces you need to examine the product for visible contamination such as slugs and caterpillars.

Foods should not be handled unnecessarily by foodworkers. The use of utensils like forks and tongs should be the normal way food is handled. The use of disposable plastic gloves can be worthwhile provided the gloves are changed between different tasks e.g handling raw and cooked meats. Also ensure that hands are washed frequently even if plastic gloves are used extensively. This is necessary as hands perspire a lot while in gloves and perspiration can leak out onto foods carrying bacteria onto foods and surfaces etc.. Latex gloves should not be used in food premises as they usually have talcum powder on the inside of the glove which subsequently becomes air borne when they are being removed and also there is now a school of thought that suggests that some people can be physically intolerant of latex rubber in their environment.

Cooking

If you were asked to stick your hand into an oven at 100°C or a container of water at 100°C for 2 seconds, which option would you choose?. Personally I would go for the oven. This is because I would be considerably less likely to burn my hand in the oven as air is a much poorer conductor of heat than water. The same is true in cooking. Cooking products in an oven takes longer than cooking in boiling water.

If foods are to be cooked in an oven then they should only be cooked when the oven is preheated to the cooking temperature to ensure that the heat penetrates the food as quickly as possible. This in turn means that the food is in the danger zone for a shorter period of time.

When cooking meat or similar products try to keep the size of the meat joints below 2.5 Kg or 100mm maximum diameter if possible. This will ensure that heat penetration will take place quickly and evenly. Larger portions may easily result in the outside of the product being burnt while the inside still remains uncooked. Foods, as mentioned previously, must be cooked to a centre temperature of at least 74°C for two minutes. Verify this temperature by using a probe thermometer.

Poultry carcasses should ideally not be stuffed at all as otherwise poor heat penetration may result in the centre of the food remaining insulated from the cooking process.

In microwave cooking ensure that manufacturers' instructions are followed properly and that food is either agitated or allowed to stand for the recommended time so that all parts of the food are properly cooked. Remember that it is heat that will kill any bacteria present not the microwaves.

Always have sufficient cooking space to cater for peak demands as otherwise you will be forced to cook food too far in advance of it being needed for consumption.

Serving and Holding food after cooking.

Once food is properly cooked then the safest time to eat it is directly after it is cooked. This assures that if bacteria are reintroduced onto the food that they will not have time to grow and also that spores cannot germinate. Foods which are ready to eat should never be handled by foodworkers hands. Only clean serving tongs and utensils should be used.

If you cannot serve the food immediately after cooking then you should either keep it hot at a temperature of at least 63°C or alternately cool the food quickly and refrigerate it. Cooling should ideally be done in a rapid chill cabinet and take no longer than 90 minutes to bring the food down to a temperature suitable for placing in the refrigerator, coldroom or freezer as appropriate. Liquid foods can more easily be cooled if emptied into shallow trays. While exceptions are allowed to enable small quantities of foodstuffs to be out of refrigeration or hot holding for up to 90 minutes while awaiting service this should only be practised where no suitable alternative is available. In my view, it is rare that a suitable alternative cannot be made available if there is the will to give highest quality service.

If food is to be reheated all parts of the food should be brought to a temperature of at least 70°C. Foods must not be reheated more than once and thereafter if they are still not consumed they should be disposed of.

Remember that when we refer to temperatures for food, we are not referring to the temperatures of the holding cabinets, ovens, refrigerators etc. we are deliberately referring to the food temperature. Temperature gauges are extremely useful for giving us an indication of temperature levels in a particular mechanical or electrical appliance but it is the temperature of the food, not the appliance, that is most important.

For example, the temperature of a hot holding cabinet might have to be at 70°C so as to hold the food at a temperature of at least 63°C. This is because all holding appliances loose heat to the outside of the unit on a continuous basis.

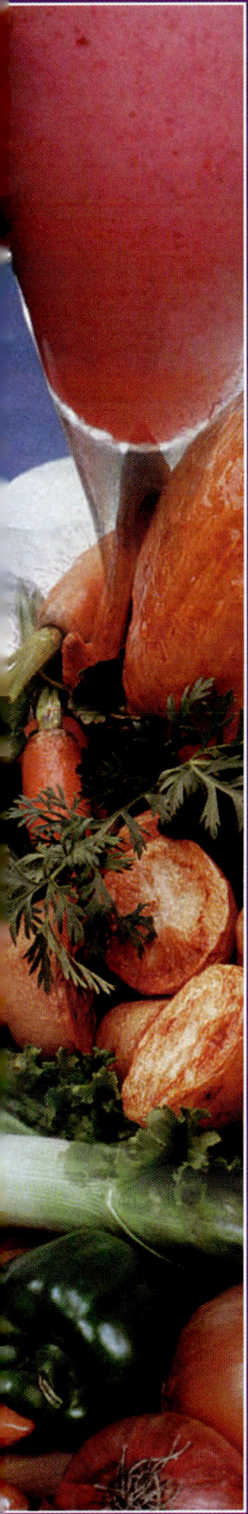

CHAPTER 5

PERSONAL HYGIENE

Nobody can know for certain that you practise good personal hygiene except yourself. Your customers trust you to keep your bugs to yourself.

5

Personal Hygiene

We have already seen that bacteria are, for all practical purposes, everywhere. They are introduced into the kitchen in a number of ways. For example, they are already on foods which are brought into the premises, they are on work surfaces and wipe cloths, they are carried in by pests such as flies and, very importantly, they are carried in by ourselves - the people who work in the establishment.

Our bodies are covered in bacteria, most of which help maintain the health of our skin and prevent skin infections. And bacteria are not just on our bodies - they are also in our bodies, particularly in the mouth, nose, throat and intestines. They are present in high concentrations in infected cuts, spots or other disorders.

Most of the bacteria in our intestines are very necessary to maintain a healthy intestinal environment. Many people react unfavourably to oral antibiotics because the necessary bacterial population in the gut are partly killed off, followed by subsequent thriving of unfavourable organisms such as certain yeasts. You can now buy "capsules of bacteria" from pharmacies which replace normal intestinal bacteria.

However, not all bacteria in or on our bodies are beneficial and many can cause food poisoning when introduced on to food by bad personal hygiene.

Human Sources of Pathogenic Bacteria

The main source of pathogenic bacteria is probably our intestines, which can carry such food poisoning bacteria as E-coli, Clostridium perfringens and Salmonella. And remember, we don't have to be ill with food poisoning to carry these dangerous germs. In fact, you could well be excreting these organisms on an on-going basis when you go to the toilet - without even knowing it. This is why employers are advised to have potential food workers questioned about previous illnesses to determine whether they could be carrying any dangerous organisms and so pose a special risk to food.

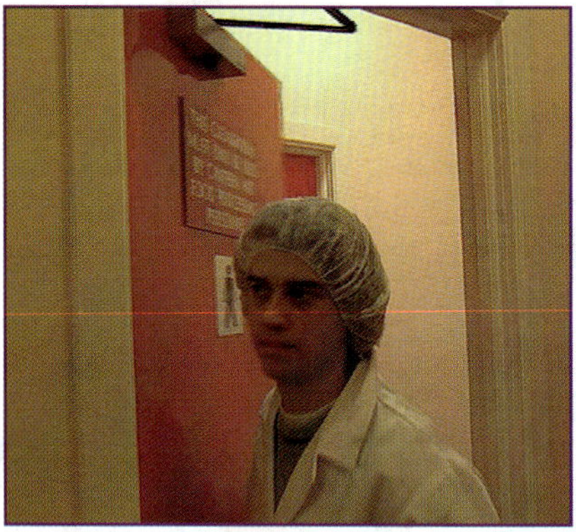

It is a criminal offence for food workers to neglect washing their hands properly after using the toilet.

So, how can dangerous bacteria be transferred on to food? The simple answer is that our hands come into contact with faecal material when we use the toilet.

Toilet paper is very porous and when we touch soiled toilet paper our hands are contaminated by dangerous germs, even when soiling is not visible. If contaminated hands are not properly washed, we will carry these germs back to food storage and preparation areas where they will be introduced onto food.

Now imagine for a moment that you enter a restaurant for lunch. The cooked ham in your salad has been handled by a food worker who used soiled toilet paper and so has literally transferred faecal material on to your food. It doesn't even bear thinking about! As previously mentioned, your customers place a trust in you and expect you to handle their food hygienically. If from this handbook each and every food worker clearly understood the need for proper hand washing, especially after going to the toilet, and put this understanding into practice then that achievement alone would have made this publication worthwhile.

Remember also that it is your legal responsibility to do this. Food Hygiene legislation requires you to wash your hands, and forearms if necessary, as often as may be required, and always after visits to the toilet. Failure to do this is a criminal offence.

Many food poisoning outbreaks are caused by people failing to wash their hands after using the toilet. Tracing food poisoning outbreaks can entail screening all food staff working in a particular establishment. This screening can reveal that a particular food worker carries the same bacteria which caused the outbreak (bear in mind that a food poisoning bacteria like salmonella can have 2,000 different types and screening will show the exact type).

From this screening it can be concluded that a particular food worker did not wash his hands properly after visiting the toilet and went on to handle food, thereby being the direct cause of the outbreak. Imagine how you would feel if that food worker was you. It is bad enough if somebody becomes ill as a result of your failure but what if somebody dies?

The importance of proper hand washing at all times, but especially after a visit to the toilet, cannot be over stressed. I have used the term 'proper hand washing' deliberately because it is not enough for a food worker at any time just to wet their hands hurriedly and call that proper hand washing. Proper hand washing entails using liquid soap and a nailbrush to wash your hands thoroughly, especially around the fingernails, between the fingers and the backs of hands.

Hands

Our hands are used for many and varied tasks throughout each day - from bringing in fuel for the fire to changing babies' nappies. A food worker's hands must be cared for almost like those of a surgeon.

Nails should be clean, short and free from varnish which might chip off into the food or obscure any dirt under the nails. Food workers should never bite their nails because this transfers possibly dangerous germs from mouths to hands and

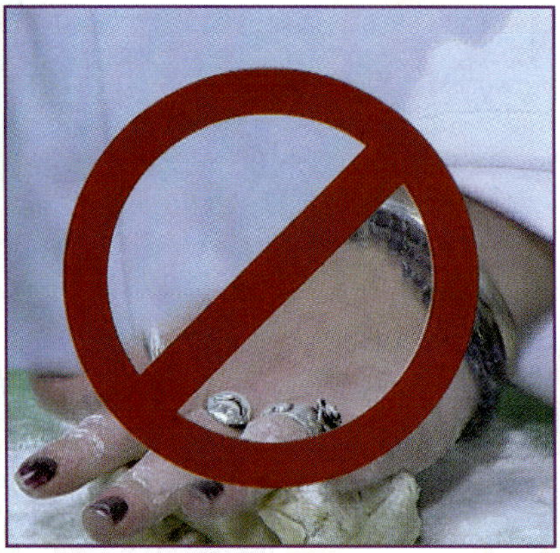

subsequently to food. Rings, watches or other jewellery should not be worn on hands or wrists. Apart from harbouring germs, there is always the risk that such items could break, causing parts to fall into food. A food worker's hands should be washed frequently throughout the day simply because, as mentioned earlier, bacteria grow on our skin where they are constantly deposited by perspiration from deep within the pores. However, there are certain times when hands must be washed, such as:

1. After visiting the toilet.
2. After any unhygienic practice such as picking your nose, touching your mouth, picking at spots, touching your hair, handling a handkerchief, or smoking.
3. When you first enter a food preparation area to start work or after a break period.
4. Between different tasks, especially after handling such items as raw meat, vegetables, money, cleaning cloths or materials.

To ensure that hands can be readily washed at these times, suitable and serviced wash-hand basins must be provided in all toilets, changing areas, kitchens, food preparation and retail areas. Remember that even washed hands can still carry dangerous germs so the use of disposable gloves is to be encouraged. However, such gloves can themselves become contaminated on the outside and are capable of transferring germs from one food to another or from other materials or surfaces. They should not be used for any unhygienic practice.

There is no substitute for not handling food at all where this is possible. Full use should be made of serving tongs, forks and spoons. Again, Food Hygiene legislation states that a food worker 'must not unnecessarily handle food.' Foods to be consumed without any further cooking should not be handled at all by foodworkers' hands.

An example of this would be slicing meat from a slicer directly on to your hands instead of on to a plate, plastic bag or greaseproof paper.

Individual food workers (not just the proprietor) have been prosecuted under this requirement. Food workers must also ensure that when off duty and when engaged in particularly dirty jobs, such as weeding the garden or working on a farm, their hands must be well protected with gloves.

Upper Respiratory Tract

The nose, mouth and throat harbour pathogenic germs too. These germs can be transferred to food when we sneeze near food or indeed laugh or talk too close to food or when we spit or touch our mouths when smoking. A high percentage of people - particularly those working in larger establishments - carry the food-poisoning bacteria staphylococcus aureus in the upper respiratory tract. In addition to this means of transferring pathogenic bacteria and viruses on to food, they can also be transferred by tasting food using our fingers or by not changing tasting spoons after each use.

Cuts and Skin Infections

Cuts are a special food contamination risk. When the skin is cut or broken, foreign bacteria immediately penetrate the skin, reaching the flesh, where they have an ideal opportunity for growth and multiplication. The body's defence mechanisms go into action straight away and the battlefront between our 'good guys' and the foreign 'bad guys' can produce pus and infection. Pus may only be there in invisible quantities but it can carry millions of dangerous germs.

It is essential, therefore, that food is protected from these bacteria. A cut, particularly on our hands, must first be cleaned up and then covered with a waterproof dressing, preferably blue in colour so that it can be readily seen if it falls into food. Be careful to ensure that the dressing is waterproof for many of the so-called waterproof bandages on sale only ensure that the sticky part is waterproof while the actual cut-covering material may still allow the infection to seep from the cut on to food.

Apart from protecting food from a cut, the waterproof dressing also protects the cut from any incoming dirt or infection.

Special precautions must be taken when a food worker suffers from such infections as acne or whitlows, as well as dermatitis, eczema or psoriasis. Obviously, suitable first aid kits are essential in any food business.

Tummy Bugs and Other Infectious Diseases

When a food worker has some kind of tummy upset, particularly when it involves vomiting or diarrhoea, that person has an obligation to refrain from working with food until such time as one is satisfied that the

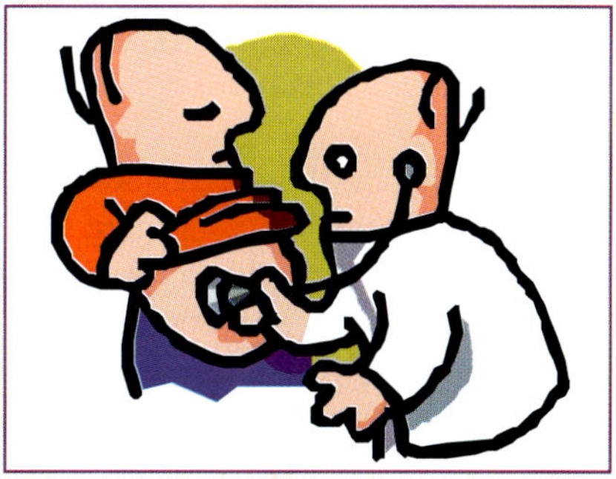

You should not work with food while you are suffering from diarrhoea or vomiting unless you first check with your doctor or Health Board. You must also inform the proprietor of the food business if you are ill in this way.

upset does not pose any risk to the food. Any person with food poisoning or gastroenteritis obviously poses a real threat to consumers by transferring large numbers of dangerous bacteria or viruses to food. Even after the acute phase of vomiting and/or diarrhoea has passed, the sufferer can go on to become a carrier of the organisms for some considerable time after an apparent recovery.

A food worker must always inform the proprietor of a food business that he/she may be suffering, or have suffered, from possible gastro-enteritis or food poisoning. The proprietor, manager or supervisor must then in turn inform the Health Board. The Health Board will then decide what action is necessary and if they consider there may be any risk to food, the worker concerned will be taken off work, or at least off working with food. Subsequently, the food worker will be screened to determine when it is safe to resume work.

Similarly, if any person living with or having intimate contact with a food worker, is suspected of having food poisoning or gastro-enteritis, then the food worker must take the same steps as if he/she had the symptoms personally. Again, the Health Board will decide on the course of action required in each case. All good food business proprietors will interview every new food worker to see whether he/she could be a carrier of any disease or condition that might in any way be a risk to food.

There are other infectious conditions such as types of infectious hepatitis, tuberculosis and similar conditions that may also indicate that a foodworker should not work with food at that particular time. The moral is that if you are in doubt you shouldn't take the risk but instead check it out with a medical doctor or Health Board.

Outer Clothing

We have already said that food workers should keep themselves generally clean and this entails taking a regular bath or shower and frequent changes of underclothing. Outer clothing must also be clean at all times.

A food worker must change into clean protective 'food worker clothing' on arriving for work. Personal lockers should always be available in a place away from any food room and private enough to permit changing of clothes. Under no circumstances should street clothing or shoes, handbags etc. be stored in or near a food room.

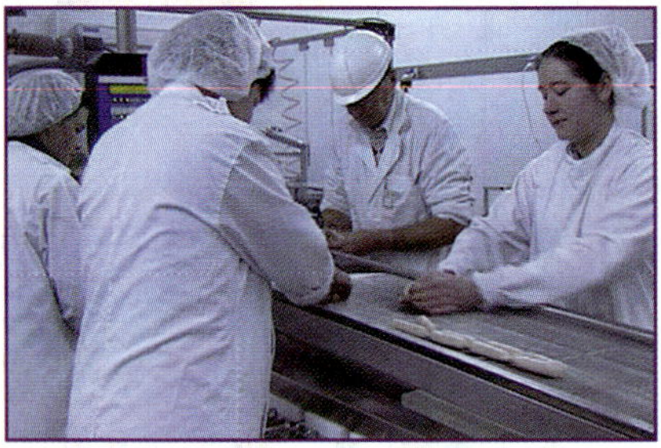

Hair should be covered in a manner that prevents loose hairs falling into food.

Suitable, clean outer clothing must be available to each food worker and this should also include suitable head gear which will not only cover the top of the head but enclose all the hair as well.

Proprietors should always consult food workers on their choice of uniform and head gear in particular, at the same time ensuring that the clothing is fashionable. It is a continual uphill struggle to get food workers to wear head gear which they don't like and resent wearing.

Aprons should be provided to protect outer clothing where the work may be particularly messy. Food workers must resist the temptation to put on protective clothing and then cover this with a jumper or cardigan. Extra clothing should be worn inside the protective clothing rather than outside. External food worker clothing should be washable, have no external pockets, be fastened only by Velcro, studs or zips and be bright in colour. Suitable safety non-slip footwear must also be worn.

If, as a food worker, you find yourself engaged in non-food work, such as a nurse's aid in a hospital or nursing home, or on toilet-cleaning duties, you must have a separate set of protective clothing for these purposes. Staffing should be arranged to render changes of duty unnecessary, except in unforeseen circumstances, such as when a staff member becomes unexpectedly ill.

Legal responsibilities of foodworkers

Remember that a foodworker includes a proprietor of a food premises, an employee in that premises and any person working in a premises where food is processed, prepared, stored, distributed or offered for sale or supply. In this chapter, you have seen that foodworkers have many responsibilities to ensure that they minimise the risk to consumers of the food that they produce, prepare or sell. These responsibilities are not just moral obligations but they are legal responsibilities too. You have to know what good food hygiene and personal hygiene are before you can practise them.

This is why it is now also a legal obligation that foodworkers are properly trained in this respect. Every foodworker is legally obliged to be trained to carry out the tasks for which they are responsible in the full knowledge of how they can prevent risk to consumers. It is now possible that staff from the statutory body who inspect your premises can ask you directly what kind of food work you are engaged in and how you ensure that this work is carried out hygienically.

For example, it would not be unreasonable that an Environmental Health Officer, or equivalent, might ask foodworkers to illustrate that they know all the important temperatures for the safe storage and preparation of food in the premises, if they have responsibility for these tasks. While the individual foodworker bears the responsibility of having and practising good food and personal hygiene, the proprietor of the food business must ensure that they receive this training by whatever means necessary.

The Health Boards provide some training in food hygiene and personal hygiene but often they do not have the resources to provide as much training as is needed. It is clear that the ultimate responsibility for training of foodworkers must rest with the food industry itself. This may involve bringing in private consultancy companies to provide training for staff or alternatively training a small number of quality control staff to provide training on an on-going basis within the food business.

The legal responsibilities of a foodworker could be summarised as follows:

Ensure that you are adequately trained in, and practise, good food hygiene and personal hygiene so as to perform the tasks for which you are responsible in the food premises in a manner that will safeguard the health of consumers of the food that you prepare or sell.

Visitors to food premises

Legislation also requires that any person who is in a food premises, for whatever reasons, such as customers, visitors or maintenance personnel, must also ensure that they do not do anything that might contaminate food. This might include, for example, spitting, smoking, or handling open food unnecessarily, in the case of customers. Maintenance personnel must ensure that they do not contaminate food either personally or by the work they are doing when in the premises. Persons who are not wearing proper protective outer clothing should not be permitted entry to food preparation areas.

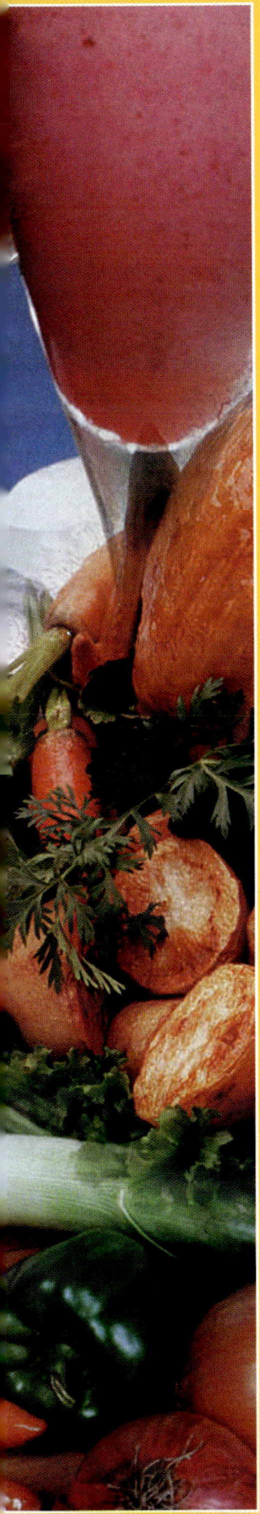

CHAPTER 6

DESIGN AND LAYOUT OF FOOD PREMISES

A little forethought in the design and layout of food premises can ensure that your business operates efficiently with less labour and effort.

Design and layout of Food Premises.

It is much more desirable to design food premises properly before the commencement of the food business rather than subsequently having to carry out expensive renovations to meet the necessary statutory and operational standards. A premises that is well designed and laid out will ensure not just greater efficiency of operation but also ensure that it is easier to clean, maintain and provide an environment where food can be hygienically stored, prepared and served more easily. Food staff are more likely to have a better sense of pride and general well-being in a good premises. It makes sound economic sense to invest a lot of resources in ensuring that you "get it right first time".

Remember that certain categories of food premises such as restaurants, take away food premises, hotels, butchers, delicatessen counters, food manufacturers or distributors must be registered with the Health Boards before the premises is allowed to open for business. The proprietors of these businesses must apply to the Health Board for registration at least one month before the proposed opening date.

The Health Board will then view the premises and can refuse registration if it is unsuitable. Alternatively, the Board can grant the premises a maximum of two periods of provisional registration of up to six months for each separate period. Otherwise the premises may be granted full registration if it is of a suitable standard.

Provisional registrations are only granted where the premises is of a high standard but not in full compliance with the food control legislation. The provisional registration periods enable the proprietor of the premises to carry out works necessary for the proper operation of the food business. However no provisional registration is granted should there be any risk to the safety of customers.

Layout and design.

It is not possible to deal with layouts for all food premises in a handbook such as this. However we will briefly examine the design and layout of catering premises and the principles used can be applied generally to other types of food premises.

The standards set out in the National Standards Authority of Ireland publications for food premises should always be consulted when you are designing a food premises. At the time of publication of this book the following standards have been published:

NSAI Standards

(a) I.S.3219:1990 Codes of Practice for Hygiene in the Food and Drink Manufacturing Industry.

(b) I.S.340:1994 Hygiene in the Catering Sector.

(c) I.S.341:1998 Hygiene in Food Retailing and Wholesaling.

(d) I.S.342:1997 Guide to Good Hygiene Practise for the Food Processing Industry in Accordance with Council Directive, 93/43/EEC on the Hygiene of Foodstuffs.

NSAI, Standard Sales Office, Glasnevin, Dublin 9. Tel: 01 807 3878.
Fax: 01 807 3841.

There is, of course, no better mechanism for identifying the structural and layout requirements for food premises than by consultations with your Environmental Health Department or the appropriate statutory authority responsible for your premises.

As mentioned earlier, areas such as goods reception, dry goods store and vegetable store should be towards the rear of the premises. This not only ensures easy access for deliveries, but also prevents unnecessary soiling of kitchen or retail sales areas due to contamination from unwashed vegetables or soiled boxes. It also ensures that delivery personnel do not have access to food preparation areas.

A **staff changing room and toilet facilities** should be located as near as possible to the yard area or other staff entrance, so that employees can change into clean work clothing before entering food preparation areas. It is very important that food staff do not share toilet facilities with non-food staff such as customers.

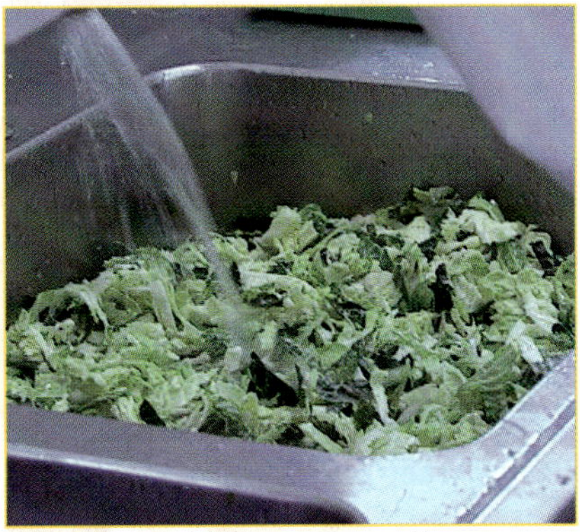

Vegetable-wash sinks must not be used for any purpose other than vegetable washing.

A **wash-hand basin,** liquid bactericidal soap with dispenser, a nail brush and hand-drying facilities should be located at the kitchen entrance and within or immediately adjacent to food preparation areas. Wash hand basin water supplies should preferably be foot or knee operated. Obviously, all toilet areas must have suitably serviced wash hand basins also.

The **cleaning store and mop sink room** should also be located as near as possible to the back yard or rear staff entry point.

The size of the kitchen depends on the volume of business and the range of products handled. The following guidelines on kitchen layout should be borne in mind, but the District Environmental Health Officer should be consulted on the requirements for particular premises.

Vegetable wash could be sited within the vegetable store, but if this is not possible, the wash and preparation area should at least be close to the store, to prevent unwashed vegetables contaminating clean areas.

The vegetable preparation area should be identifiably separate from the rest of the premises, although any separating walls need not necessarily be to ceiling height.

However, the area should be designed so that it can be hosed down during cleaning. Washing or storing vegetables beside other foods will result in bacteria from vegetables contaminating those other foods, as well as worktops and equipment with which vulnerable foods come into contact.

A pastry and dessert preparation area, with its own work surfaces, should be provided in one of the cooler parts of the kitchen. Desserts, creams, etc. are very vulnerable high-risk foods and provide an ideal medium for germs to grow quickly under suitable conditions.

Raw meats should be prepared on separate work surfaces, using equipment which is not used for other foods. It has been shown how raw meats can be heavily contaminated from the slaughterhouse. Anything with which these meats come into contact will become cross-contaminated - surfaces, equipment, other food, personnel and so on.

Cooked meats must also have their own preparation surfaces and equipment. Many cooked meats are eaten cold, so that the entire loading of bacteria could be ingested without further cooking or re-heating to kill them.

It is recommended that each of the above areas are easily identifiable to every food worker in the premises. To assist in this it is recommended that separate colour coding of utensils and chopping boards should be used. The recommended colours are:

- Blue - Fish
- Red - Raw meat
- Green - Salad and fruit
- White - Dairy and bakery products
- Yellow - Cooked meats
- Brown - Vegetables

Pot wash may be provided by automatic pot-washing machines in larger establishments but even smaller premises must have at least two deep sinks for the exclusive use of pot washing. This facility is often located adjacent to the cooking area where dirty pots are generated. Proper pot-racking facilities are essential. Apart from having preferably jointless, hygienic floors, potwash areas should also be slip resistant.

Dish wash is best located close to the service area or dining room, so avoiding the need to carry dirty dishes back through the kitchen. It also allows clean dishes to be readily available for plating up or for table laying. Automatic dishwashers are essential in modern premises but remember that these must always be supplemented by the traditional double-bowled sink for manual dishwashing, with a hot detergent wash in the first bowl and a very hot rinse in the second. Manual dishwashing must be available in case of dishwasher malfunction or a power cut.

The **still room** must always be provided as close as possible to the dining area.

Items of **cooking equipment** should be grouped together to provide efficient extraction of heat, steam and cooking odours. All such equipment must be overhung with a stainless steel canopy served by drip channels, fluted grease filters (which are more easily cleaned than the wire mesh type) and a mechanical extract fan of sufficient size. Cooking equipment should preferably be sited on an 'island' or central location in the kitchen, rather than adjacent to walls, so that there is no obstruction to cleaning. The use of wheeled cooking equipment is to be encouraged.

Service fridges, those holding vulnerable food likely to be required within a short time for cooking or serving, should be located near the dining area, holding milk, butter, orange juice, wines and the like. Similar fridges near the cooking area (but not too close) will avoid frequent trips to and from the coldroom. Unless this procedure is followed, vulnerable food could be left close to the cooking area, in the warmest part of the kitchen, for perhaps several hours, resulting in the growth of dangerous levels of bacteria.

Good **lighting** is essential in any food establishment for a number of reasons:

1. It enables all areas to be readily seen and shows up those requiring cleaning.
2. Food deliveries can be properly inspected.
3. All foods can be effectively examined to ensure that they are not visibly contaminated with soil, insects or other pests.
4. If a dangerous object, such as a thumb tack or a piece of glass, were accidentally introduced to the food area, good lighting will help to ensure that it can be seen and removed.
5. Labels on foods and cleaning materials are easier to read.
6. Fewer accidents are likely to occur.
7. The presence of rodents or other pests will be more readily apparent.
8. A well-lit environment is conducive to better working and increased diligence.

It is preferable to have a good mixture of artificial and natural light. Remember, too, that all artificial lighting should be enclosed in shatterproof diffusers, so that if a bulb or tube breaks then fragments of glass cannot fall into food.

Ventilation

Good ventilation is very important in all areas because:

1. Germs need moisture for their growth, so the more moisture removed from food preparation and storage areas the better.
2. Excess heat and steam are removed at source, so that a cooler environment is provided for food thereby minimizing bacterial growth. Employees who work in a cooler, less humid environment are more diligent, more productive and suffer less fatigue.
3. Excess steam will also result in a need for more frequent decoration and increased operating costs.
4. Dry foods such as flour will spoil if good ventilation is not provided.
5. Good ventilation in toilets and toilet lobbies prevents foul odours permeating the rest of the building.
6. While it is often felt, from a sales viewpoint, that some cooking odours attract people to an establishment, bear in mind that excess cooking odours can be nauseating to customers.
7. With smoking becoming less socially acceptable, it is important to remove smoke from 'smoking permitted' areas. Even where smoking is still widely permitted, such as in pubs, customers appreciate an efficient ventilation system.

Localised mechanical extract ventilation must always be provided over heat-and-steam-producing equipment. The canopy serving such areas should be high enough to ensure comfortable head-clearance. Fluted filters must be provided on the canopy in order to prevent grease being drawn into the ducting and on to external walls and roofs at the point of discharge.

Of course, there is little point in providing good extract ventilation unless suitable intake ventilation is also provided. Care should be taken in the placing of inlets for ventilation to ensure that they are most likely to take in air of the cleanest quality available in the area.

Grease-laden ducting is a serious fire hazard. Canopies should also have suitable drip-channels, preferably discharging into a small retention cup at one corner to facilitate regular cleaning and a rounded grease channel is easier to clean than a V-shaped one.

Wire-mesh grease filters are, thankfully, becoming less common. They pose an onerous cleaning problem, with many premises possessing two sets, so that one can be left for steam-cleaning while the other is in use. I have seen cases where pieces of wire mesh have fallen into food as the result of continuous cleaning with caustic solutions.

Many people fail to place canopies over such items as dish-washers and still-room boilers, or at least site them close to good air extraction points. I know of many premises where this factor was not considered at the planning stage, resulting in costly intervention at a later date.

Work Surfaces

There is no substitute for good quality stainless steel work surfaces. Over recent years, local production of high-standard stainless steel products to customers' specifications has been readily available around the country. Most of these engineering concerns also provide a design service.

Extensive use of melamine-faced (Formica topped) chipboard worktops is diminishing

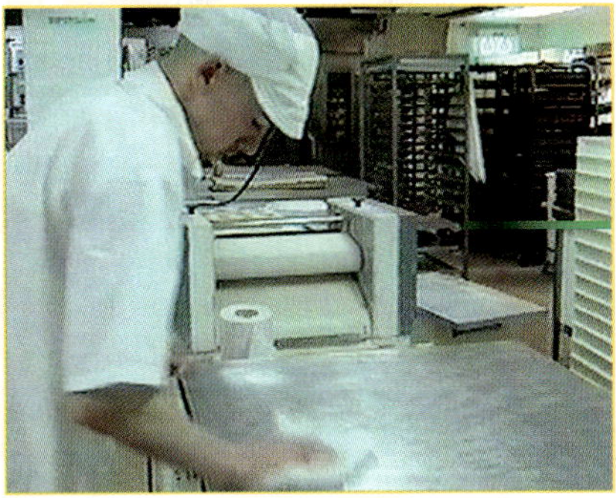

as people appreciate the durability and cleanability of stainless steel. Of course, stainless steel is expensive in the first place but it is considerably cheaper in the long term.

Many food establishments now use mobile work surfaces with lockable wheels. This not only simplifies cleaning worktops and adjoining walls and floors, it also permits relocation of work surfaces to improve workflow. Cooking equipment is also wheel-mounted for the same reasons.

Floor Surfaces

Floor surfaces should be easy to clean, impervious, durable and slip-resistant. These requirements pose something of a dilemma, because 'easily cleanable' and 'slip-resistant' are seemingly contradictory terms. Floors which are easy to clean are usually smooth and extremely slippery when wet, whereas slip-resistant floors have a rough surface which makes them very difficult to clean.

What is needed, therefore, is a surface which provides a good balance between these two factors - in other words, smooth and slip-resistant. PVC safety flooring is widely recommended for this purpose. Many kinds of floor tiling and sheeting meet these requirements, as do a number of the modern floor-coating paints.

Altro safety flooring, a slip resistant sheet vinyl, is widely used in commercial and institutional kitchens.

It is important that floors should only be laid by professionals. I have seen far too many proprietors of food businesses saving money by doing such work themselves and ending up having to spend three times more to get the job put right in the end.

Where floor paints are concerned, use caution when dealing with inexpert companies, with little or no back-up services. Many such firms come and go each year, leaving proprietors of food premises with inferior products which will not stand the test of time. One should deal only with the more reputable companies which have been around for a long time. While no firm can be regarded as being entirely safe from business failure, there is a greater chance that the long-established firm will still be in business in a few years' time.

Joints between floors and walls should be coved, or rounded, for easy cleaning. If floor tiles are to be laid they should be bonded only to smooth, even floors, otherwise they will inevitably crack, creating additional health and safety hazards. Steel tiles must be laid in certain cases where metal-wheeled trolleys are used, such as on the approach to ovens. With any floor covering, it is essential to check with the suppliers or manufacturers that it is suitable for the purpose intended, as some floor surfaces are badly affected by certain foods, especially those of an acidic nature.

Walls

The final finishing on internal walls should be applied to a very high standard and be smooth and joint-free. Wall tiles which have been processed to withstand high temperatures can often be used, although more and more authorities are insisting that walls are finished in suitable high-quality special non-porous wall paints or hygienic wall cladding that can withstand high-pressure hosing during the cleaning process. These measures are also favoured by EC guidelines.

Altro Whiterock wall and ceiling cladding provides an hygienic, easily cleaned and impact resistant surface for commercial and institutional kitchens.

Even with high-standard wall tiles, grouting in the joints can be semi-porous and where it is not flush with the tile surface the consequent recesses between tiles can be dirt and germ traps. It is important, of course, that the plaster in new walls and concrete in new floors be allowed to dry out thoroughly before any paint is applied. Similarly, it is imperative that walls or floor surfaces are not contaminated with oil or grease before any final finish is applied, as this will result in poor adhesion and subsequent flaking of paints.

Wall surfaces behind cooking equipment, wash-up sinks and worktops should be clad in stainless steel and professionally fixed to the wall, with no unhygienic seams. These areas are subject to extreme variations in temperature, heavy wear and tear, with frequent heavy impact from pots and pans. Panels of stainless steel to a height of 18in is normally considered sufficient above work surfaces but having work surfaces and cooking equipment away from walls is better still. Alternatively, work surfaces can have a lip of a suitable height at the rear to protect the wall.

Ceilings

Normal plasterboard ceilings are quite suitable for most food premises as indeed are most washable types of suspended ceiling. Opinions vary as to the surface to be put on the plasterboard - some feel that ordinary flat emulsion paint is sufficient where there is adequate ventilation. It is agreed that this allows the surface to 'breathe' and delay any condensation if, for example, a dishwasher is opened.

Other opinions suggest that a gloss paint be used to make it more washable although, in this case, condensation may occur more quickly. Similarly, it can be argued that emulsion paint can be re-applied more easily than gloss paint and is, therefore, likely to be applied more frequently. Again, there is a significant movement towards the use of proprietary ceiling cladding, particularly of the joint-free, easily cleaned variety. The colour of ceilings should be bright to allow for maximum reflection of light.

Water Supply

As already mentioned, only water of suitable "potable" quality may be used in food premises. If you are unsure of the quality of your water supply you should seek clarification from the Health Board or Local Authority. Alternatively, you could arrange to have the water tested

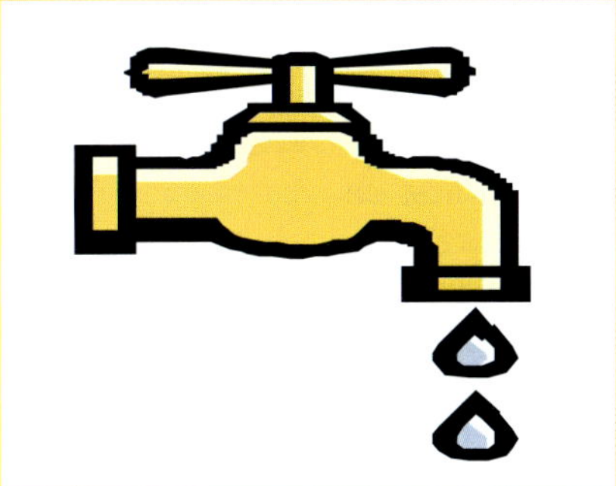

Do you know if the drinking water to your premises is safe? If not, have it checked.

independently. Ensure that only water directly from the rising main is used for direct consumption, food preparation, or washing utensils and equipment. Also ensure that the same direct supply feeds any ice making installation. Always see that roof tanks for water storage are properly covered to prevent contamination by insects, birds, rodents or other pollutants.

Drainage

All food premises should be connected to properly constructed, regularly maintained drainage systems. Most drainage systems in urban areas connect to the public sewer while in rural areas some food premises connect to their own private treatment plants or septic tanks. Generally septic tanks are not considered suitable for any business larger than a cottage-type process and even in this instance it depends on the type of food business involved.

Internally there must be no direct access or ventilation to foul drainage systems within a food premises. Connections to the foul system must only be made in such a manner that guarantees foul water or foul matter cannot back-flow into the premises. Access chambers to drainage systems often provided in very large premises must be pressure sealed. Air or water breaks must be provided between sinks, washers etc. and the foul drainage systems.

Pipe joints for the drainage system under the floor or in the ceilings of food premises must be pressure sealed and sited to minimise the effects of any drainage maintenance that might have to be carried out from time to time. Proper, easily understandable drainage plans of the premises should be kept at the food premises.

Waste and Refuse Disposal

All food establishments generate waste which varies from food containers, boxes and wrapping materials to food waste, debris and liquid waste.

Retail premises generate a substantial amount of cardboard and wrapping materials which can be extremely bulky. Many supermarkets encourage customers to use empty boxes to contain their purchases, a form of recycling that is to be encouraged because it can conserve other materials. However, storage of these boxes close to the point of sale must be orderly and the boxes themselves must be free from contamination which could taint or otherwise contaminate foodstuffs.

This means removing any boxes which contained detergents or other chemicals and soiled boxes must not be used. I once witnessed fresh cream cakes being wrapped in a box soiled from raw chickens!

Boxes and wrapping materials can be baled and firmly secured in small compactors to reduce their bulk and to limit the space required for storage.

Tightly enclosed skips with compactor fittings are ideal for larger premises. Large skips without compactors are less suitable but are acceptable, provided they are pest-proof. All refuse storage receptacles and stores must also be pest-proof.

Manually filled skips should be provided either with a platform for easy access by staff or alternatively placed at a lower level than the surrounding yard. In the latter case, safety rails should be in place to prevent accidents.

Properly sealed skips and bins ensure your waste does not unduly attract pests to your premises.

All external bins should be of substantial, durable construction and be kept firmly closed by a lid-securing latch or handle. Bins should preferably be kept in a pest-proof external store or raised on a platform above ground level to facilitate cleaning. All refuse stores or containers should be located a reasonable distance from the actual food premises to minimise the possible effects of odours or any temporary breakdown in pest-proofing measures. All such storage areas must have washable concrete floors, preferably sloped to drainage, and should be within reach of a water hose equipped with a high-pressure jet.

Skips and bins must be cleaned after emptying. It is essential that refuse is removed from the premises as frequently as possible. If one relies upon local authority refuse collection, it must be remembered that responsibility for frequency of collection rests ultimately with the individual establishment. Private arrangements for refuse collection must be employed if public services are insufficient.

Internal short-term storage of refuse is necessarily acceptable, provided that it is hygienically contained. There are slightly conflicting views on the type of container that should be used for internal refuse storage. One view holds that they should be pedal-operated covered bins or bags while another view is that they should be open containers or open frame held bags. The argument for the latter option is that food workers often contaminate their hands when putting refuse in lidded containers even if they are pedal operated. Whatever type you use, the most important consideration is that the containers are emptied frequently.

Much food waste and debris can be disposed of by means of a garbage grinder/macerator attachment to a sink unit which is normally located close to the point of dish or pot washing. Some Local Authorities are now becoming more concerned about the use of these devices as they can have an adverse effect on the public drainage system. Any establishment discharging a liquid waste that may contain grease must provide a good-quality grease removal trap which must be regularly cleaned and serviced. Similarly, if significant quantities of starch or vegetable debris are generated, then sedimentation traps should also be provided.

As will be outlined later, the hygienic storage and disposal of food wastes is one of the most important control measures in pest-prevention.

Food stalls

Food vehicles is the term used for vehicles that are used simply for the transportation of food while the term "food stall" is used to describe a vehicle or structure from which food is sold by retail. The stall may vary from a travelling retail shop to a chipper van. Some of these stalls, particularly the stalls on which food is prepared or cooked, must be licensed each year with the local Health Board. Legally, it is an offence to operate one of these stalls without a licence and because of the mobile nature of stalls, Health Boards tend to prosecute the stallholders of unlicensed stalls without notice.

The principles of food storage, preparation and service are no different in food stalls than in food premises. However, by their nature, structural surfaces will be different but nonetheless must be easily cleanable, impervious and durable. All licensable food stalls must have hot and cold water on tap, wash up sinks, wash hand basins properly serviced, first aid kits and adequate ventilation where appropriate. The cab area must be separated from the rest of the vehicle and there must be a reliable source of power to operate refrigerators, freezers and cooking equipment. There must also be suitable methods of retaining waste water from the sink and wash hand basin.

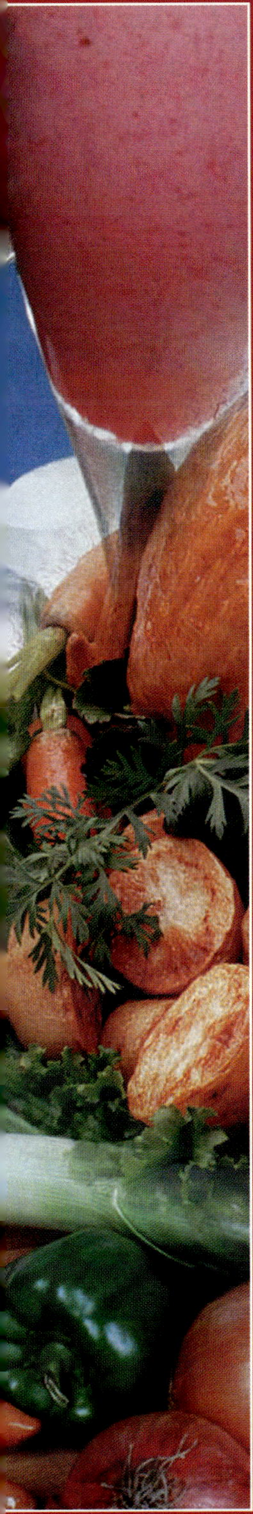

CHAPTER 7

PEST CONTROL

Pests carry disease. Preventing pests entering your premises is always better than trying to eradicate them after they have gained entry.

7

Pest Control

Keeping pests away from foods is essential in any establishment. Common pests include rodents (rats and mice); insects such as flies, bluebottles, cockroaches, food mites; birds, cats and dogs.

First of all, let us examine why we are concerned with keeping such pests away from food:

1. Many of these pests may carry disease themselves or can transfer diseases from sewers, dumps, refuse and excreta. Diseases carried by rodents include Weils disease and salmonella. Flies vomit digestive enzymes on to food before they eat it.
2. They can result in the spoilage and therefore wastage of much food due to their droppings, urine, dead carcasses, gnawing of foodstuffs and generally by their very presence on or near food.
3. They can cause considerable structural damage. Rats, for example, must gnaw to survive. They have incisor teeth which grow up to four inches each year and if allowed to grow to this extent, the rat will eventually die. Continuous gnawing keeps the teeth short and sharp. They will gnaw electric cables, lead pipes, doors and all kinds of timber and plastics, causing fire, flooding, electrocution or even explosions.
4. They can cause upset and revulsion which can actually lead to subsequent phobias and even physical symptoms such as vomiting.
5. Rodents and other pests can fall into open water storage tanks in lofts.
6. Rodents can, in certain rare circumstances, bite people.

Signs of Pests

The presence of pests such as dogs, cats, flies and birds is usually obvious, particularly as they can be seen during day time. However, many pests, like rats, mice and cockroaches, normally emerge only at night, so the absence of sightings is not sufficient proof of their absence. Periodic night-time inspection of premises, some time after the lights are switched off, can visibly reveal the presence of nocturnal pests.

PESTS CARRY DISEASE

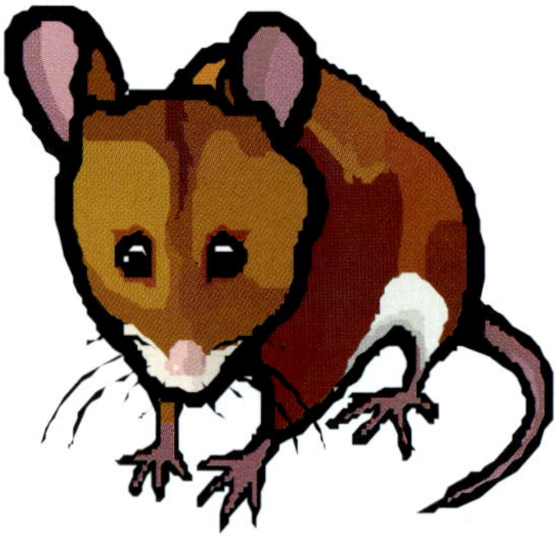

Other signs to notice include:

Rats & Mice

a) Droppings

b) Gnawing of food, parts of the structure, containers, or paper

c) Dead carcasses

d) Particular smells associated with mice, especially in enclosed spaces, and the foul smell of a decomposing carcass

e) Rodents have an oily fur which discolour the likes of skirting boards and ceiling joists if the rodents run along these over a period of time.

f) Paw marks in dust

Insects

a) Dead carcasses

b) Pupae or egg sacs

c) Webbing from various insects like moths

External Attractions

Pests, like humans, need food, shelter and warmth, some seeking these necessities most particularly in winter time, especially rats and mice.

As with all aspects of food hygiene, prevention is better than cure. The first step in prevention is to make premises less attractive to pests. The means to this end include:

1) Keep vegetation around premises short, neat and well maintained in order to minimise cover for insects and rodents.

2) Keep site tidy and ensure that all outbuildings are well maintained and protected against access by pests.

3) Keep all drains properly sealed, including manholes, gulleys, and vent pipes.

4) Most importantly, keep refuse bins and bags tightly sealed against insects and rodents. Skips and bins must have tight fitting lids or otherwise, like bagged refuse, be kept in a pest-proof externally located refuse storage area. All areas used for refuse storage should have concrete floors or paving. The concrete should be laid to a fall to facilitate the area being hosed down regularly. Bins should be stored on a washable stand at least one foot off the ground to provide easier access for cleaning the surrounds.

Rodent Entry to Buildings

There are many means by which rodents may gain entry into the premises. These include:

1) Open doors; this may seem very obvious but it is surprising how often doors to food premises are left open for long periods during the day or night. External doors should be kept closed as much as possible and fitted with strong self-closing devices. Alternatively self-closing and tightly fitting swinging transparent-type plastic doors could be provided.

2) Even small spaces beneath doors can give ready access to rodents. There are premises where considerable sums are spent on a rodent control contract while rodents have full access beneath external doors. As rodents also gnaw the bases of doors, it is recommended that a nine-inch high metal kick-plate be affixed to the base of the door. Doors should be tight fitting, with thresholds which are level and as close as possible to the bottom of the door. Metal threshold bars are useful for this purpose and in difficult situations hard rubber or plastic edging on the base of the door can be worthwhile, as long as they are stiff enough to prevent rodent entry and are well maintained and replaced as necessary.

3) Rodents are good climbers so even windows, particularly low-level ones which are left open at night, can be an open invitation to rodents.

4) One of the most common access points for rodents is around waste and service piping. Many plumbers fit outlets to sinks, wash-hand basins, and WCs without sealing the hole in the wall around the pipe. Where a cavity wall is involved, remember to seal the space on the inside wall as well, for there may be rodents in the cavity. Of course, it is not only the spaces around waste and water pipes that might allow rodent entry but also around any services below or above the ground, such as telephone, electricity or TV cables.

5) Rodents can even gain ready access to new buildings, since these are unlikely to be rodent-proof before completion. Building workers should avoid leaving food debris on such premises and ensure that all drains are sealed off at the end of each working day. All pointing in blockwork should be completed, leaving no gaps for rodent entry, particularly at lower levels. Similarly, all spaces around service pipes and cables passing through ceilings should be sealed, especially where they enter attic spaces.

6) Ventilation openings under floors, in walls or for coldroom motors should be sealed off with proper wire mesh.

7) Rodents can enter in food packaging or containers, which is one reason for thorough inspection of all incoming goods.

Rodent Refugees inside Buildings

Even if all preventive precautions fail, measures can still be taken inside the building to make it difficult for rodents to remain undetected for any appreciable time.

1) All foodstuffs should be properly enclosed at night in rodent-proof containers or rooms, and refuse removed at the end of each day.

2) Goods should be stored in an orderly manner off the floor,for ease of cleaning and early detection of rats and mice.

3) 'Dead' spaces which are poorly boxed off or are inaccessible for inspection and cleaning should be eliminated.

4) Since rodents need water, all possible source of supply should be protected, including roof tanks.

Elimination of Rodents in and around premises

There are several options for eliminating rodents but there is no better means of control than prevention. Some elimination methods include:

1) Poison baiting - The use of any poison within food premises carries the risk of contaminating food. Strict care must be taken to ensure that poisons are treated as already outlined for other dangerous chemicals. Many Environmental Health Officers believe that because of the food contamination risk, rodent bait should not be laid in food storage or preparation areas. Their argument is that the layout and design of the premises should reveal the rodent presence at an early stage and that more active elimination procedures should be taken immediately. Poisons have the disadvantage, of course, that the affected rodent may die on the premises. Many of the anti-coagulant poisons make rodents thirsty and cause them to seek water - hopefully outside rather than in your roof tank.

   Poison laying in food premises should preferably be done by professionals. Externally laid rodent poisons must be protected against access by children, birds and animals.

2) Trapping - Spring loaded snap traps or cage traps can be very useful, especially for mice. Mice are inquisitive creatures and will come to a trap readily, while rats are more suspicious by nature and may take several days to accept a new object in their environment.

   The advantage of trapping is that the dead rodent can be suitably removed. Where there is major infestation, trapping may only be effective initially since other rodents may quickly become aware of the danger, having seen the fate of earlier victims.

3) Cats - The use of cats for rodent control in and around a food establishment is not acceptable as they can be as much of a hazard as rodents. The cure can be worse than the disease.

Insect Entry to Buildings

1) Flies, bluebottles and other insects gain entry to a building through open windows and doors, especially if refuse is stored too close to the building. The obvious solution is to keep windows and doors closed as much as possible or ensure that they are properly screened.

2) Proper insect screens must be fitted on openable windows and ventilation grills in food preparation and storage areas. Internally, food should be kept covered as much as possible to protect it from the chance contamination by insects. However, even if food is covered insects can still cross contaminate food by alighting on work surfaces, crockery etc..

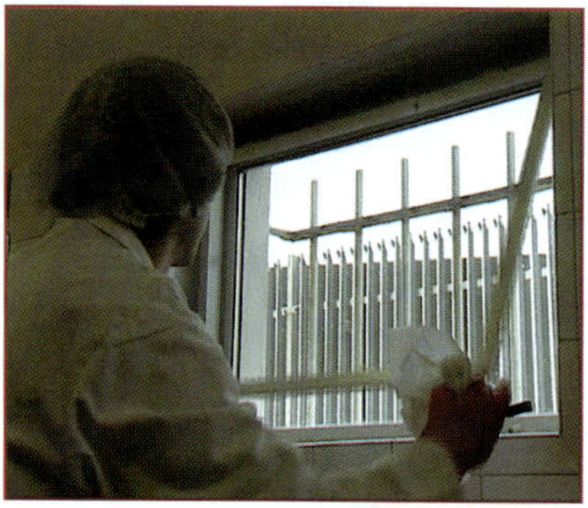

All openable external windows should be fitted with suitable insect screens.

3) Obviously, insects can gain access to premises by the same means as those used by rodents. However, due to their smaller size and the fact that they are far more likely to infest food, even penetrating packaging, the inspection of incoming foods and those ready for use becomes even more important. It is essential that foods which are susceptible to insect infestation, such as flour, rice and other cereals, be inspected more frequently. Flour should be regularly checked for flour mites by levelling part of the surface with the back of a spoon and leaving it to stand for about 20 minutes. If the levelled surface presents a ruffled appearance it is likely that the flour is infested with flour mites.

Insect Refugees within Buildings

The same refuges used by rodents are also available to insects. However, due to their small size, insects can more readily gain access to pipe ducting, open food packaging and containers. Cockroaches, particularly, seek cover in or near sources of heat. Foods such as flour and dried soups must also be kept in dry, cool conditions which help reduce the multiplication rate of infesting insects. All false panels and inaccessible areas should be removed.

Elimination of Insects within Buildings

Electrocuting devices are generally helpful in destroying insects, although their effectiveness varies greatly according to the model and its proximity to fluorescent lights which appear to have just as much attraction. Recent research has suggested that some of these devices occasionally cause the victim to explode, sending pieces up to 20 feet away and possibly into food. Some companies now sell a model which only briefly stuns the insect, which then falls on to sticky paper impregnated with insecticide on which the unfortunate creature comes to a 'sticky' end.

It must be remembered that all such devices need to be maintained, tubes replaced and dead flies and other insects must be removed frequently in the interests of food safety.

The old style sticking tape suspended from the ceiling can be useful, although rather unsightly, but needs regular replacement.

The disadvantage of sprays is that the insect can fall into food and, of course, some sprays are not suitable for use in a food area.

Strips of insecticide-impregnated materials which claim to release the insecticide slowly over a couple of months also have the disadvantage that affected insects can fall into food. Furthermore, if premises have a high ventilation capacity, the effectiveness of these materials can be severely diminished.

Cats and Dogs

Staff in food premises frequently feed stray cats and dogs. This only encourages the animals to stay around the premises more and they often come inside the building

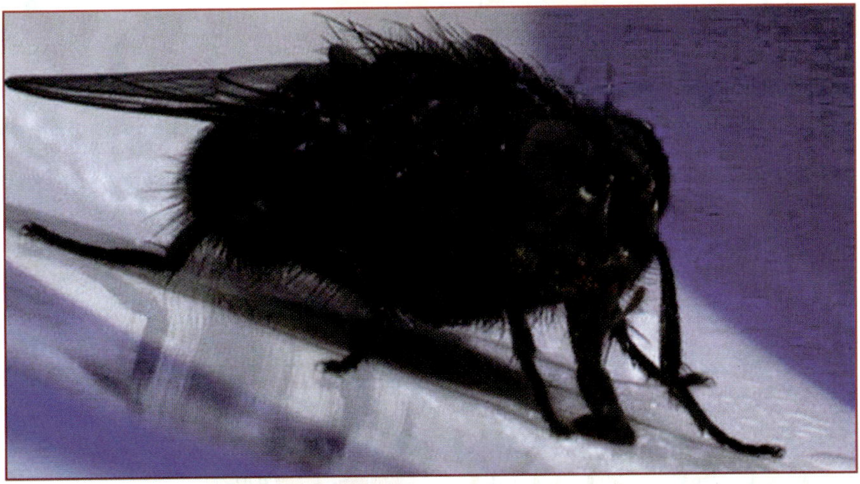

The common house fly vomits onto food, so as to help its digestion, before eating it.

when doors etc. are left open and unattended. In domestic premises that may be involved in preparing or selling food it is not acceptable that family pets have access to food areas. Exceptions need to be made for the presence of guide dogs on food premises as these dogs are trained in a special manner.

Birds such as sparrows can be a particular problem with certain food premises such as bakeries. The proper control of refuse storage, the screening of openable windows and doors and the loading of food vehicles within enclosed areas can help to control birds.

Hanging plastic curtains or air current barriers can be helpful.

If more assistance is needed, a specialist pest control company should be engaged.

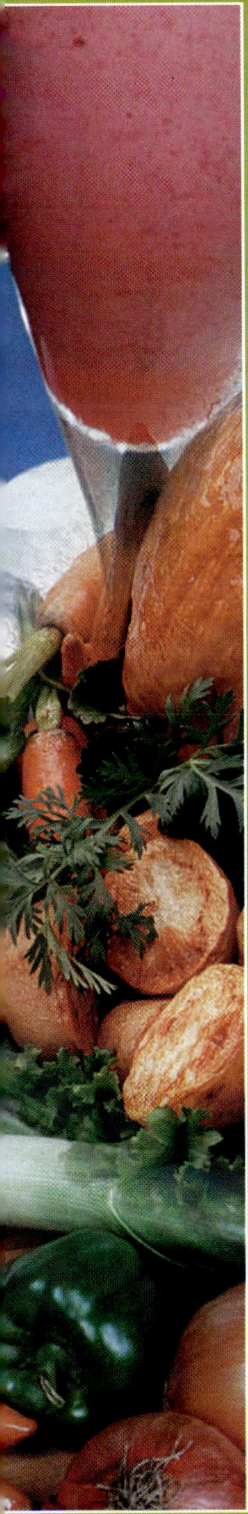

CHAPTER 8

CLEANING

The task of cleaning is often incorrectly viewed as being of lower importance than other food work. However, just because premises look clean doesn't automatically mean that they are safe.

Cleaning

Cleaning - the method by which we remove food residues, dirt and grease - is obviously an essential part of food hygiene. While we regard proper cleaning as common sense and an essential practice, let us examine more closely why it is so necessary. Dirt has many components, such as dead skin from our bodies (over half of all house dust is dead skin!), food waste and debris, moisture, and above all germs - some of which may be harmful.

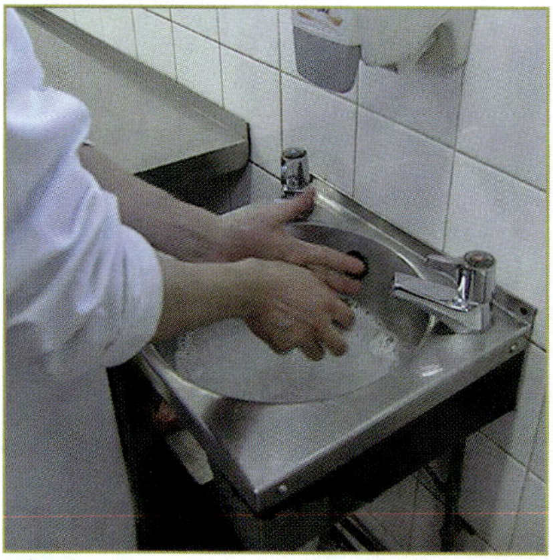

Wash your hands after handling cleaning materials.

Obviously, nobody wants to consume another person's dead skin any more than they wish to get food poisoning from dirt getting into their food.

Dirt in a food establishment is particularly undesirable because it presents an ideal medium for bacteria to grow. As we recall, bacteria need warmth (found in all commercial food premises), food (which makes up a large proportion of any dirt in food premises), moisture (normally present in dirt) and time to grow.

Thus cleaning is needed to:

- Reduce the risk of cross contamination
- To prevent food spoilage and food poisoning
- To ensure a safer working environment
- To promote a favourable image to customers
- To comply with the law

It is essential that dirt is quickly and regularly removed from food premises. It stands to reason that soiling, food spillages or food smears are removed most easily at the time they occur. Dried-in dirt and dried-in food spillages are relatively difficult to remove. It is important on the other hand to remember that just because something looks clean that does not mean that it actually is clean. A steel worktop wiped with a dirty cloth can look quite clean but will still have what could be called 'invisible dirt' and perhaps colonies of dangerous bacteria. When cleaning some parts and facilities of food premises, we need to effect a standard of cleaning that will reduce the number of bacteria to safe levels.

Cleaning is achieved by using:

1) Physical energy
2) Chemicals
3) Heat energy ... most of the time by using hot water (remember it must be potable water for cleaning purposes).

Physical Energy

Basically, physical energy means using 'elbow grease' or scrubbing with mops, brushes and mechanical jets or cleaners.

Chemicals

Chemicals employed to assist cleaning in food premises include:

-Detergents
-Disinfectants
-Sterilants
-Sanitisers

Detergents

A detergent is a chemical which allows water to soak right into dirt and grease, thereby allowing them to be removed more easily. If you pour water and oil into a glass you will see that water and oil do not mix. This failure to mix is due to a barrier between the two liquids caused by 'surface tension.' Surface tension is a force occurring on the surface of a liquid which behaves like an elastic skin. Detergents help to break down this barrier between the two compounds. It is important to remember that detergents do not kill bacteria, but by helping to remove the dirt, detergents allow a high proportion of the bacteria to be removed with the dirt as well.

In using detergents properly and effectively, it is important to remember the following points:

a) There are detergents which are not suitable for use with equipment and surfaces that will subsequently come into direct contact with food - so make sure that the detergent you use is suitable for the purpose. Many chemical companies producing detergents and disinfectants are only too delighted to visit your premises to advise on what detergents are suitable for your needs. They may also provide instruction cards on each product which can be handed to whoever is doing the cleaning. These cards give brief information under such headings as:

- Purposes for which the product is suitable
- Concentrations at which it should be used
- Any special safety precautions

b) It is essential that detergents are used in concentrations as directed by the manufacturer. Many premises waste significant sums of money by the inappropriate and improper use of detergents. Remember also that detergents get used up during use and need to be replaced. Solutions containing used up detergents should not be topped-up but replaced altogether.

c) Detergents are not for consumption so it is essential that they are thoroughly rinsed off any surface which may come into direct contact with food or food material.

Disinfectants

A disinfectant is a chemical which kills most bacteria and reduces their numbers to safe levels, but it does not kill all bacteria (a chemical which kills all bacteria is known as a sterilant.) Again, the following points must be borne in mind when using a disinfectant:

a) Disinfectants should only be used on surfaces that are already clean. They do not work effectively on dirty surfaces.

b) As with detergents, there are specific disinfectants which are suitable for use in any food storage or preparation area. It is, for example, necessary for the disinfectant to be non-tainting, easily rinsed off and reasonably non-corrosive. When choosing a disinfectant for use in contact with surfaces that come into contact with food, be sure to choose one which is suitable for such use.

c) Disinfectants must be used properly and that includes using the proper concentration and observing the required contact time (the length of time necessary for a disinfectant to be in contact with bacteria in order to kill most of them and reduce their numbers to safe levels).
Disinfectants used in concentrations that are too weak will fail to reduce bacterial contamination to safe levels, and those which are too strong result in unnecessary wastage. Where too weak a solution is used, it gives a false sense of security for it is presumed that an item is properly disinfected when in fact it is not.

d) Bacteria can grow in disinfectant solutions which have been used up or have become stale. At this stage the use of such a solution actually spreads rather than kills bacteria.

e) It is worthwhile to periodically change the types of disinfectant used because bacteria in a certain environment can become immune to a disinfectant which has been in use in the same area for a long time. This is particularly true of places such as hospitals.

f) Consider carefully whether the use of a disinfectant is appropriate. For example, there is no advantage in using disinfectant on the floors of kitchens or food storage areas. Firstly, the floor does not come into contact with food and, secondly, shortly after treatment the floor will be walked upon and the bacteria reintroduced. Normally, where crockery, cutlery and pots and pans have been thoroughly washed in either a double-bowled sink or in a dishwasher where the rinse temperature is high enough (82°C) then there is no need to use a disinfectant. However, because larger items of equipment and worktops cannot be washed by these methods, disinfectant is necessary when they are being cleaned, i.e. after each use in the case of a worktop. Again, remember to follow the instructions carefully and rinse off the disinfectant when necessary.

g) As with any chemicals, take proper safety precautions when using disinfectants, particularly when they are in concentrated form.

h) Unfortunately there is no easy manner of knowing when disinfectants are used up.

Sanitisers

These are combined detergents and disinfectants and as such they help both remove dirt and also reduce the numbers of bacteria. It is generally accepted, however, that they are somewhat less effective in their disinfecting role than disinfectants on their own. However, they still play a useful role in cleaning.

Sterilants

These are chemicals that destroy or remove all living micro-organisms. Sterilisation is not practical or necessary in food premises as surfaces etc. will become recontaminated easily.

Heat

Whenever possible, heat should be used to kill bacteria and thereby effectively disinfect. It is preferable to put small items of equipment such as cutlery into very hot water (82°C or higher) for a few minutes rather than leave them in a solution of disinfectant.

Heat assists in the removal of dirt and the efficiency of detergents. It is easier to remove dirt with a solution of hot water and detergent than with cold water and detergent. Most chemical cleaners lose a considerable percentage of their effectiveness when used with cold or cool water and such use proves very wasteful.

Wipe Cloths

Apart from the direct means of cleaning we should not overlook the wipe cloth, an important and universal cleaning aid which, when incorrectly used, can be a source of cross contamination throughout any food premises. As already stated, bacteria need food, moisture, warmth and time to grow.

Often used to mop up food debris, a wipe cloth is almost always wet, is usually stored at room or warm kitchen temperatures and is often left lying around for long periods of time. So it provides the ideal place for bacterial growth, including dangerous bacteria. Since bacteria are transported from one place to another, a wipe cloth can easily provide this means of transportation.

The following important factors in wipe cloth usage must be borne in mind:

1. Single-use disposable wipe cloths or paper cloths should be used and disposed of immediately after use, whenever possible.
2. Wipe cloths must be easily identifiable for different purposes. Floor cloths, for example, should be of different material to those used in the raw meat section. Similarly, this latter cloth should be different to the cloth used for surfaces in the cooked meat area or for wiping dining room tables. Such separate use ensures that cloths do not carry bacteria from one surface to another or from one food type to another.
3. When a wipe cloth is used, it should be properly washed out and left for laundering or at least placed in a covered container of a suitable disinfectant if it must be reused.
4. As with all cleaning aids, cloths used in toilet areas must not be used in any other area.
5. Remember that wipe cloths also contaminate hands, so don't forget to wash your hands after using a cloth.

6. Don't confuse dish-drying cloths with wipe cloths. Dishes should, of course, be air-dried in any event.

Cleaning Programmes

We take it for granted that such items as crockery are cleaned after each use.

Similarly, work tops must be cleaned after each use and floors cleaned after a spillage and after each meal service. When we are engaged in a task of preparing foodstuffs then the task is not finished until we have cleaned up afterwards. As we know, the sooner cleaning is effected the easier it is and the less chance for bacteria to grow. The principle of "CLEAN AS YOU GO" is worth putting into practice.

However, in any food establishment there are items and areas that need regular cleaning but the appropriate intervals necessary for such cleaning may not be so apparent. Obviously, any part that looks dirty needs cleaning immediately. Food storage presses, wall areas, fridges, ice-cream dispensing machines etc. may be overlooked or not cleaned as regularly as necessary.

It may also be unclear as to whose responsibility it is to clean certain areas or equipment and very often what is everybody's responsibility ends up being nobody's responsibility. In each establishment, individual food workers or cleaners must be given direct responsibility for cleaning each piece of equipment. In this way the food worker or cleaner is held legally responsible for carrying out this task and if the job is not done properly then everybody knows who is at fault.

All food premises must have a cleaning schedule or programme. Such a schedule stipulates

1. Each item or piece of equipment or area to be cleaned
2. How often cleaning should take place
3. What cleaning agents are to be used and the dilution rate
4. The procedure for cleaning
5. Safety instructions to be followed
6. The person who is responsible for the cleaning
7. Who is responsible to check that the cleaning has been properly carried out
8. How all areas and facilities are to be cleaned and how often.

This prevents areas or facilities being missed or forgotten or not being cleaned as often as necessary. This should also include "deep" cleaning which concerns such items as grease traps and grease filters. Many establishments have a daily or weekly written cleaning programme where the person or persons responsible for cleaning have to confirm on a chart that the area or item has been cleaned by them.

Cleanability of Premises and Equipment

The design of premises and the surfaces used should be given careful consideration from a cleaning point of view. As already mentioned, walls and floors should have easily cleanable surfaces, preferably with coving between floors and walls. Ledges and unnecessary decorative work should be avoided.

Work surfaces should not be easily scored and none should have joints or edging materials which trap dirt. Worktops and counters, as well as any equipment which may be used for "dirty" jobs or give rise to spattering, should be located away from walls, preferably in the centre of the floor. All equipment, including cooking facilities, should ideally be movable to allow proper cleaning with the minimum of effort.

Even though the more suitable work and wall surfaces such as stainless steel are expensive, they are more economical in the longer term. Thankfully, most modern food equipment is designed with cleanability in mind but one should still ensure that all equipment purchased have no areas which are inaccessible for cleaning. Wooden surfaces and chipboard have no place in modern food premises, with the possible exception of a properly-constructed butcher's block.

Floor Cleaning

Some important points to remember about floor cleaning include:

1. Wet floors can be slippery and dangerous. Insofar as it is possible and practical, try to confine floor cleaning to the times when premises are less busy. Always place "slippery floor" signs in prominent positions to warn employees and the public alike.

   Place good quality, heavy, readily washable matting inside external doors, particularly on wet days, to prevent both dirt and water being carried into the premises. The use of PVC safety flooring is advisable.

2. As mops can spread dirt as readily as pick it up, ensure that mop heads are properly washed, disinfected and dried after use.

3. Try as much as possible to prevent spillages on to the floor. How often in fruit and vegetable shops do we see foods such as grapes over-stacked on shelving and frequently falling on to the floor, to be trodden in. When spillages do occur, remove them as soon as possible.

4. A mop-sink should be available in every establishment and under no circumstances should a wash-up sink be used for cleaning mops or for the direct filling of mop buckets.
5. Many people seem to have an aversion to picking things up off the floor. Cleaners sometimes brush an item such a cigarette packet right through the premises rather than pick it up and put it in the bin. Similarly, where hosing of a floor is appropriate, a similar item might be hosed continually from one end of the premises to the other - what a waste of time and energy.
6. Don't forget areas you can't easily see, such as beneath shelving in a retail grocery - please take the trouble to clean these areas as well.
7. Separate cleaning mops, cloths and cleaning water solutions should be used for toilet cleaning. Failure to do so will result in toilet germs being carried into food areas.

Dishwashing

Crockery and cutlery come into direct contact with food and with our mouths. Consequently, they can transfer germs to food and from one consumer to another. When using a cup you don't want the mouth infection or the flu virus from the last customer to be transferred to you!. Particular emphasis must be given to cleaning these items. In our houses most of us have a single kitchen sink with one bowl. What, then, is the best way to wash dishes in this?

Firstly, in all cases, dishes should be cleared of as much food residue as possible by scraping or indeed sometimes by rinsing prior to washing up. This initial rinsing needs to be under flowing warm water where possible. However, if you have a greasy plate, this rinsing will not be very effective, so you might consider wiping the grease off as best you can with a disposable paper towel.

From a common sense point of view the cleaner dishes should be washed first. The scraped dishes are then immersed in the bowl which should contain very warm water (just bearable to hands wearing rubber gloves) and suitable detergent. Dishes should be well scrubbed with a suitable brush or pad. They should then be visually inspected and if found to be satisfactory they can be rinsed under flowing hot water.

In the case of a commercial kitchen, dish washing is carried out either in a mechanical dishwasher or double-bowl sink. The preparation remains the same for either form of washing. However, in the double-bowl sink, the second sink is used for rinsing off the detergent and for disinfecting the dishes with hot water (at least 82°C). For this purpose, the hot water in the second sink, while not at boiling point, should be so hot that even with gloves, the hands cannot be immersed in it. Obviously, dishes must be immersed using a wire or plastic tray that fits properly into the sink bowl.

An alternative to using hot water for disinfecting purposes is the use of a suitable dish disinfectant or sanitizer in warm water, in which case the manufacturer's instructions should be followed. Dishes should then be left to air dry. If dishes do not air dry then the rinse water was not hot enough. Drying cloths usually make dishes dirty rather than clean.

Mechanical dishwashers should be used according to the manufacturer's instructions, with suitable detergents, rinse aids, salts etc. as appropriate. Mechanical washers operate on the same principle as the double-bowl sink. Again, careful inspection must be carried out after washing and any soiled articles returned for further washing.

Check mechanical dishwashers to ensure that they are operating satisfactorily. It is important that the jets are not blocked, that adequate temperatures are being reached in the different cycles, that the dosage rate for the detergent is appropriate, and that the rinse aid is being dispensed as necessary.

In all cases articles such as dishes, pots, pans and glasses should be washed as soon as possible after use, when food debris is easier to remove. A common complaint when washing glasses is that they are stacked when hot after washing. This can result in glasses sticking together and having to be prised apart with the hands, thereby contaminating the glasses again.

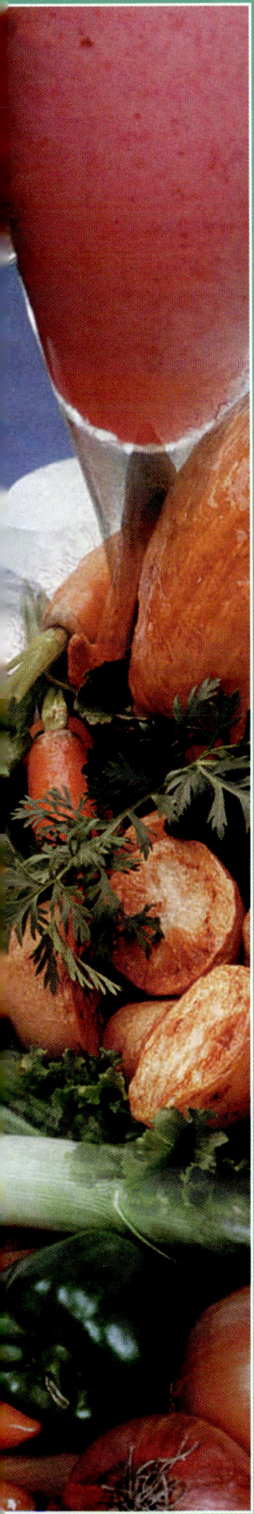

CHAPTER 9

AN INTRODUCTION TO HAZARD ANALYSIS CRITICAL CONTROL POINT

The title may seem a little daunting but Hazard Analysis Critical Control Point (HACCP) is no more than a common sense way of keeping food safe

An Introduction to Hazard Analysis Critical Control Points Systems

During the American space programme, it was essential that the astronauts would be guaranteed that they would not suffer food poisoning during any space mission. It's bad enough having food poisoning when your feet are firmly on the ground but just imagine what it would be like to have diarrhoea in space! So the NASA authorities in conjunction with some of their contractors devised a system of food safety which would minimise the risks of this happening. They called this system Hazard Analysis Critical Control Point (HACCP).

Don't be put off by the jargon-type name because like most jargon, the process it describes is not as complicated as it first seems.

Irish and European Union legislation now requires each commercial food business to develop and implement a HACCP, or similar type plan for their food business.

What is HACCP?

HACCP is a system used by food businesses to identify steps that are critical to ensuring food safety and outlines a manner in which the critical steps can be controlled so as to reduce the risks to health from food. It is not a system that will guarantee that the food is absolutely safe but it will minimise the risk.

When we are looking at what HACCP is, it is important to remember that we are presuming that all other general hygiene issues such as the suitability of the structure, good quality facilities, and appropriate cleaning are already in place in the premises. HACCP is not a replacement for good general practice - it is rather an additional safeguard.

When we are speaking of reducing risks from food we need to examine briefly what kinds of hazards lead to these risks arising in the first place. They're are three main types of hazards associated with food:

Microbial hazards - bacteria and their toxins, viruses, certain moulds, parasites etc.

Physical hazards - foreign objects such as glass, metal, insects etc.

Chemical hazards - pesticides, detergents, disinfectants and the like.

One of the best ways of coming to understand HACCP is by looking at a practical example of how it can be implemented. Let us take the example of the serving of a cooked chicken which was purchased as a fresh chicken into a catering premises.

The stages involved for the production of this food would include:

Delivery - Storage in the Refrigeration - Preparation - Cooking - and Service to the customer.

So let us examine the risks involved in each of these stages and what control measures we might implement to reduce each risk.

Delivery

Hazards	Possible Control Measures
Microbial contamination	Reliable supplier and production premises
Microbial growth	Specific delivery requirements especially time and temperature
	Delivery temperature below 5˚C
	Minimise loading and unloading time
	Check delivery personnel & vehicles
	Check date codes, packaging
	Good personal hygiene and handling

Storage

Microbial growth	Keep food below 5˚C in refrigerator
Microbial contamination	Good stock rotation
	Good cleaning
	Avoid cross contamination with other foods or unclean surfaces
	Good personal hygiene and handling

Preparation

Microbial growth	Minimise time at room temperature
Microbial contamination	Good personal hygiene and handling
	Good operational hygiene
	Prevention of cross contamination
	Cleaning / disinfection

Cooking

Microbial survival	Minimise time in danger zone (5°C - 63°C)
	Pre-heat ovens
	Cook to a minimum core temperature of 74°C for at least two minutes

Serving

Microbial growth	Serve immediately after cooking
Microbial contamination	Serve within 90 minutes holding it above 63°C
	Good personal hygiene / training
	Cleaning / disinfection

You will see from the above that the main risks specifically associated with the preparation and service of a cooked chicken is related to the Microbial type of contamination. This is not to say that a cooked chicken could not be contaminated with a chemical or with physical contamination.

However, as a caterer, you would have no specific control over whether the chicken was positive for antibiotics, for example. So you would have to hope that the producer would have ensured the product to be free of chemicals and confirmed it to you in some way, such as showing you laboratory test results.

This is what is meant by choosing a reliable supplier.

You will also note from the above that there are a lot of common controls at almost every stage such as - good personal hygiene and handling, adequate cleaning and disinfection. We could refer to these as good normal practice and thereby leave them out of what is specifically critical in the cooked chicken example.

In HACCP also it is important to keep the controls you consider to be critical to a reasonable minimum as if we consider everything to be critical then there would be little point to the entire system. In the above example of the cooked chicken the three points that I would consider to be the most critical controls, in order of priority, would be;

Cooking the chicken to a minimum core temperature of 74°C for at least two minutes is the most critical control as it destroys the bacteria present.

Where the food is not to be served immediately after cooking, but some time shortly afterwards, then the food should be kept hot at a temperature of at least 63°C.

Keeping the food properly refrigerated at a temperature below 5°C so as to prevent bacterial growth and possible toxin formation taking place.

When you decide on a critical control point it is important that this point is written down and even more importantly that all food staff who may be involved with the product know exactly what the control is. Once food staff know what the control point is, it is then important that they know how they can be sure that this point has been achieved and what they should do if they find that it has not been achieved. Let us take the first critical control point mentioned above for illustration purposes.

How do we measure this control? The obvious way is to use a probe thermometer by pushing it into the centre of the cooked chicken and verifying that the temperature is a minimum of 74°C for at least two minutes. What happens if, when the control has been measured, it is found that it has not been complied with?

In our example, if the food worker found that either the correct temperature or the correct amount of time were not reached then obviously the chicken would have to be left in the oven longer until the correct temperature and time were reached. These should then be recorded on a chart which not only verifies that the task has been carried out but that it has been carried out properly. The chart should also have a space for the name of the person who probed the chicken and wrote up the chart.

You can see that it would be a great advantage if somebody alleged that they received food poisoning from cooked chicken on your premises and you could produce the chart for this particular product for the specific day that it was supposed to have caused illness.

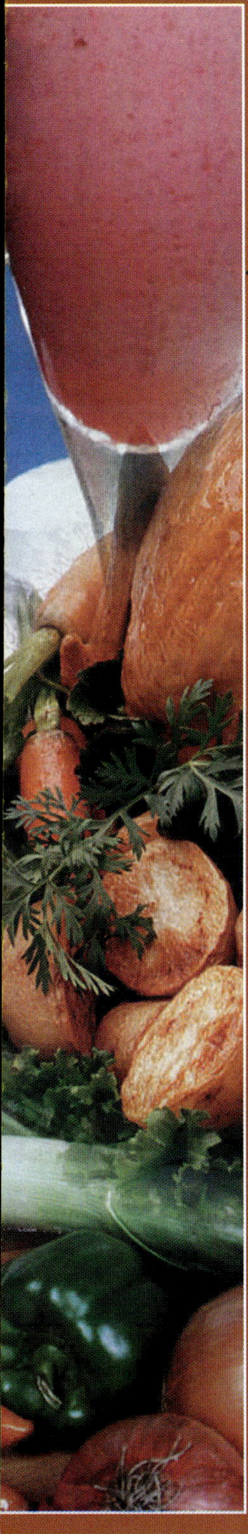

CHAPTER 10

COMMON PROBLEMS FOUND BY ENVIRONMENTAL HEALTH OFFICERS IN FOOD PREMISES

While many food hygiene problems are universal, specific problems occur in different settings including our own homes, retail groceries, butcher shops, catering and manufacturing and licensed premises.

Common Problems Found by Environmental Health Officers in Food premises

The following are some of the more common food hygiene problems which are found in particular types of premises. While these problems have been broken down into various categories, there is an obvious overlap between different types of premises and where this occurs the problem is not repeated.

A common problem which is rarely referred to but applies to all catering establishments concerns staffing levels. If premises are under-staffed then food workers who are under unreasonable pressure of work may be totally unable to give food hygiene its proper priority.

All the following problems are practical examples of principles already referred to and should be read with this in mind.

Retail Groceries

1) Frozen foods left above the loadline in freezer cabinets.

   Keep a constant check.

   Check all loading by merchandisers.

   Keep stocks of awkward-shape products such as frozen turkeys to a minimum.

   Impress upon each employee the need to rearrange frozen food when necessary, so that all items are below the load line, and emphasise the need to do this every time they pass a freezer.

   Make one employee particularly responsible for orderly arrangements within all freezers.

2) Refrigerated display cabinets and other fridges and freezers not kept at proper temperatures.

   Check all refrigerated and freezer units to ensure all sections of the units are maintaining the proper temperatures.

   Keep a constant vigil and have calibrated probe thermometers as well as indicating thermometers in constant use.

   Do not over-stock fridges and freezers.

   Keep doors of coldrooms closed as much as possible.

   Have regard to the positioning of display cabinets, avoiding draughts, sources of heat, including strong, warm lighting, all of which may increase cabinet temperatures.

   Fit plastic-strip blinds to the fronts of upright display cabinets in order to maintain low temperatures.

   Have fridges maintained regularly.

   Do not put warm food into a fridge or coldroom.

3) Foods such as cooked chickens not kept hot enough in warming cabinets.

   Ensure food is put into warming cabinets only when it is hot.

Ensure a food temperature of 63°C is maintained as a minimum and remember that this will usually mean keeping the cabinet itself well above this temperature.

4. Improper storage of the different categories of foods so that they can cross contaminate each other.

Keep high risk ready to eat foods stored separately from other foods.

Provide proper segregation of foods that are presumed to be highly contaminated such as raw meats, vegetables etc. This includes the provision of separate preparation, cutting surfaces and equipment.

5. Foodstuffs improperly labelled.

Foodstuffs such as bread, confectionery and some meat products like fresh or frozen chicken are often improperly labelled.

Retailers are responsible for ensuring that food labels are correct, and should insist that food delivered by all suppliers is properly labelled. Improperly labelled foods should be rejected.

6) Freezing of foods intended for sale as fresh.

Foods such as fresh chickens are often frozen if not sold before they come close to their expiry date: this is a very dangerous practice and a deliberate deception of customers. It also constitutes a breach of the Labelling Regulations. Foods intended for sale as fresh and handled in this manner by the supplier should never be frozen by the retailer. It goes without saying that the rare practice of defrosting frozen foods and selling them as fresh, is a potentially lethal practice and anybody found doing this should, in my opinion, be prosecuted.

7) Badly kept store areas.

It is often found that, even when a retail sales area looks good, storage areas can be a different matter altogether. Food needs just as much care in handling in storage as in the sales area.

Keep foodstuffs stored separate from other goods.

Keep the store cool in summer, warm in winter and dry at all times.

Ensure proper stock rotation.

Keep the area well lit, with stock stored off the floor.

Ensure the area is properly rodent and insect proofed.

8) No proper staff toilet

Staff working with food should have their own toilet which must be properly serviced and maintained.

9) Lack of suitable wash-up facilities.

In some retail stores it is necessary to have a wash-up sink for utensils, display trays and the like but the same sink is often used for cleaning mops which should, with cleaning buckets, have a separate sink.

Mops, buckets and brushes should also have their own separate store.

Where soft ice-cream is sold from a machine there must be suitable facilities with a deep sink for cleaning the machine.

10) Unwrapped bread and confectionery products placed where they can be readily contaminated.

Unwrapped bread and confectionery products should not be available for self service by the public but should be served only by food workers who are, of course, obliged to take all necessary precautions to ensure that items are handled hygienically.

Similarly, unwrapped products should not be displayed on top of service counters or display cabinets.

11) Improper separation of hardware items.

In shops selling a wide range of products, hardware items should be arranged in an area separate from food.

12) Sale of fuels

In retail premises which sell petrol or other liquid or solid fuels it is essential that any food worker serving these fuels wears protective clothing which is different from that worn while handling food. Close attention should be paid to hand-washing between these tasks. Better still, food workers should not handle these fuels at all.

13) Front door of premises left open.

It is difficult to insist that the door to a grocery shop be kept closed at all times, but where this is the case it does not deter customers, provided there is a prominent OPEN sign on the door. Keeping the door closed prevents dust blowing in from the street and helps to keep the shop free from insects.

14) The area beneath the service counter is often very disorderly and untidy.

15) Vegetables and milk left outside doors.

Milk must be kept in a refrigerator.

If vegetables must be placed outside the shop then they must be at least 3-4 feet above the ground.

16) Some shops sell frozen burgers, frozen fish fillets and frozen pork chops loose, without wrapping in self-service areas.

All such products must either be pre-packed or served by a food worker.

17) The growth of self-service salad and pizza counters is a cause for concern.

Customers frequently avoid plastic gloves as requested and the sleeves of jumpers and coats can often be seen dipping into various foods, particularly where the display is more than one container deep.

Droplet infection from customers sneezing near such counters can be minimised but not prevented. Customers should preferably be served by a full-time food worker.

18) Preparation of sandwiches and filled rolls for consumption off the premises.

Many retail establishments now prepare sandwiches and filled rolls for consumption off the premises, particularly around lunch-time. Where such preparation occurs it is essential that adequate space is made available for this purpose and that suitable worktops are provided and maintained for this purpose alone. Adequate equipment, wash-up, hand-washing and refrigeration must also be provided. The nature of this food preparation is much different from the normal retail business and proprietors should not consider venturing into this area without first consulting the local Environmental Health Officer.

19) Unhygienic, slippery and dangerous floors.

20) Unhygienic, cracked wall surfaces.

Butcher Shops

1) Meats not retained under proper refrigeration.

Meats should be kept out of refrigeration for the shortest possible time. It is worth noting that in some countries a temperature of below 10°C is required for the entire shop.

Remember to return cooked meats to the fridge immediately after slicing. Allowing cooked meats to stand on the slicer encourages bacterial growth.

Minced meat should be handled with particular care as it is an ideal growing medium for dangerous bacteria; meat should be minced as close to the time of service as possible but most particularly minced meat must be refrigerated as soon as it is minced. Ideally the mincer should be stored in the cold room so that any meat in the "head" is constantly under refrigerated conditions.

Remember that all meats should be kept between 0°C and 5°C.

2) Raw and cooked meats cross-contaminating each other.

Keep raw or fresh meats substantially separated from cooked meats.

Use separate work surfaces for cooked and raw meats, as well as separate slicers, knives, trays etc.

Keep decorative plastic separators well away from all foods and ensure that they are washed regularly.

Do not place such items as coleslaw and meats close together in fridges.

Keep the wrappings of foods away from unwrapped foods. We tend to forget that the outside of wrappings are often highly contaminated.

3) Cross-handling of vegetables and meat.

Over recent years more butcher shops have taken to selling vegetables as well as meat. This constitutes a serious cross-contamination risk if proper separate handling and storage is not provided.

Vegetables should preferably be sold only in pre-packed bags but if they must be handled then either encourage customers to serve themselves or wash your hands very thoroughly before going back to handling meats.

A properly serviced and more importantly - well used - wash hand basin is essential in every butcher shop.

Vegetables should be weighed on scales which are different from those used for meat, even if the vegetables are pre-packed.

4) Misuse of wipe cloths

The misuse of wipe cloths is a particularly common problem in some butcher shops.

5) Use of sawdust on floors.

There are varying opinions on the use of sawdust in butcher shops but many hold the view that it should not be used at all. Most shops manage perfectly well without it. However, where its use is acceptable to the local Health Board then the quantity should be kept to an absolute minimum. Very fine sawdust should not be used because it gets into foodstuffs too easily.

Sawdust must be vacuumed up at the end of each work day at least.

6) Labelling.

Butchers omitting to label foods such as loose sausages, which should have an adjacent sign declaring the presence of preservatives etc. where appropriate.

7) Handling money and meat.

Butchers handling money and meat and not washing their hands as appropriate. Similarly, butchers handling cooked and raw meats or vegetables without washing their hands between these tasks.

8) Windows and doors.

Lack of insect-proofing of windows and absence of fly-screen doors where entrance doors are left open constantly.

9) Hand-towels.

Using hand-towels for wiping blood-stained or dirty or improperly washed hands or equipment. A hand-drying towel in any food establishment should never be dirty. A dirty towel shows that it was either used as a wipe cloth or for drying hands which were not properly washed.

10) Failure to separate fish from meats.

11) Freezing unwrapped burgers etc. in a manner which may cause them to be contaminated.

12) Storage of food products on the floor of the coldroom.

13) Lack of suitable probe thermometers.

14) Smaller shops.

In smaller shops, where another part of the premises is used as living accommodation, the kitchen sink is often used as the wash-up sink for the butchery business. This is unsatisfactory, because the sink may also be used for such purposes as vegetable washing, household laundry and indeed may not be available for butchery use when required. Similarly, the availability of hot water for the shop may depend upon whether somebody has used all the water for a bath or some other purpose.

15) Unhygienic floors.

16) Unhygienic, cracked wall coverings.

Bakeries and Confectionery Premises

1) Some establishments fail to make their premises insect- and bird-proof. The presence of insects in bread and confectionery products is one of the most common complaints received by Environmental Health Departments. Time and time again proprietors bring an investigating Environmental Health Officer's attention to the presence of insect electrocuting devices.

These are seen as a cure-all and a sign that the proprietor is doing all that can be done. While these devices are useful, they are no substitute for screening windows and doors.

Birds such as sparrows can often gain access to bakeries, especially through open doors in the loading bay. The entrance from the bakery to loading bays should be open only while trolleys or people are passing through and the entrance door should preferably be closed automatically by sensors. Also, good waste management is essential to ensure a ready food supply is not available to feathered or furry friends, cleaning up spillages as soon as they occur.

2) Damaged wall and floor surfaces caused by steel trolleys are all too common in these premises. The proper choice of flooring material is essential and the provision of 'bump-bars' and steel corner edging is almost always necessary.

Proper steel corner edging prevents undue corner damages.

3) The control of ingredients used in relatively small quantities can be a major problem, as can flour which is stored in bags rather than in

silos. An open half-used bag often attracts insects. Inevitably, some of the bag's contents lodge in that portion of the bag which is pushed down into the food while awaiting further use. This results in further spillages onto the floor when the bag is next re-opened. The emptying of partly- used dry ingredients into suitable food bins (preferably wheeled units) or into purpose-designed hoppers, prevents all the above problems and makes food storage and preparation areas much easier to clean.

4) A significant proportion of bread products are still unsuitably labelled and the industry generally needs to tighten up in this area.

5) Failure to cool bread quickly after baking results in diminished keeping quality of the product, particularly when bread is wrapped before it is fully cooled. Also, heat given off by hot bread causes the bakery to become warmer than is necessary. Proper cooling tunnels should be used for this purpose, rather than the all too common practice of cooling in an open loading bay or outside the premises altogether.

6) Too little attention is often given to toilet facilities and the provision of essential changing rooms with individual lockers and well-maintained shower facilities. Canteen facilities, too, are often of poor standard.

7) The choice of oven design and location is also a matter which often receives inadequate attention. This frequently results in the bakery becoming almost unbearably hot and humid. Inadequate general ventilation will exacerbate the problem and can lead to extensive mould growth on walls and ceilings, spores from which heavily contaminate the product.

8) Occasionally 'home bakeries' set up in domestic premises or in converted garages, in breach of all Food Hygiene Regulations and when discovered by the local Health Board they are either quickly closed or prosecuted or forced to construct a new purpose-designed building. Special provisions for 'cottage' type businesses are being considered at the time of this book going to press.

9) Unhygienic floors.

10) Unhygienic, cracked wall coverings.

Catering premises

1) Inadequate refrigeration or refrigerators maintained at unsuitable temperatures. If any corners are to be cut in your food premises, please don't do the cutting in refrigeration.

2) Pre-cooking of foods too far in advance of consumption. This practice relies on rapid cooling, prompt refrigeration and adequate reheating - all steps which provide opportunities for preparation to go wrong and time for bacteria to multiply.

3) Insufficient staffing levels result in staff having insufficient time to practice good food hygiene.

4) Defrosting of food out of refrigeration - in the kitchen or even in sinks filled with water - thereby allowing bacterial growth which could result in cross-contamination throughout the premises.

5) Improper disposal of refuse in containers which very often are not tightly lidded to prevent pest problems.

6) Failure to rodent proof vegetables stores in particular and leaving spaces around waste pipes and beneath external doors.

7) Failure to segregate the preparation of different categories of food and provide separate equipment for each category.

8) The misuse of wipe cloths - again!

9) Unhygienic, dangerous floors.

10) Unhygienic, cracked wall coverings.

Licensed Premises

1) Insufficient, unsuitable or improperly used facilities to provide not just visibly clean but bacteriologically clean drinking glasses. Failure to clean dirty glasses can result from a number of factors, from washing in cold and sometimes dirty water, devoid of cleaning or sanitising agents, to malfunctioning glass washers or the use of unsuitable or incompatible water supplies. In many cases, while glass-washing techniques are adequate, clean glasses are either dried or polished with dirty cloths or carelessly mishandled by the rim.

2) The use of dirty ice can be a significant problem, particularly in the case of small rural premises. This can result from freezing unsatisfactory tap water in domestic freezers where the water is not suitable for direct human consumption and where the ice is subject to contamination from other foodstuffs, packaging etc. in the freezer. In urban locations where the water supply is known to be good, the ice maker may be plumbed from a roof tank rather than the correct means i.e. directly off the mains.

Moreover, ice makers are often sited in less than satisfactory store rooms or corridors and the machines omitted from poor cleaning schedules. Furthermore, drinking glasses which may be handled again and again are often deposited in ice buckets for dispensing purposes, thereby constantly transferring germs from hands to ice and finally into the consumer's stomach. Only proper long-handled ice tongs should be used.

Ensure ice is only made from water directly off the rising main and from a suitable water supply. Proper handling with long handled tongs suitably stored gives your customers clean ice.

3) Inadequate smoke extraction is all too common in licensed premises, although with increased awareness of the right of the non-smoker to be protected from the inhalation of secondary smoke, the situation is rapidly improving and one hopes this continues.

4) Inadequate attention to cleaning of toilets and the provision of suitable toilet facilities. In many establishments, especially when they are busy, staff are not made available to inspect toilets and this can result in an otherwise hygienic toilet facility becoming disgustingly dirty in a very short time.

Proprietors constantly excuse poor toilet facilities on the grounds of vandalism. I appreciate that toilets can be subject to a high level of abuse yet two premises located close together with a similar clientele can vary in standard considerably. Vandalism can be reduced by good design, where cisterns are inaccessible to patrons, pipes are concealed within or behind walls and the area as a whole is planned to prevent abuse. It is also essential that bar staff and ancillary personnel inspect the toilets very frequently and carry out necessary cleaning.

Clean toilets regularly inspected and maintained by staff show you care.

5) Inadequate cleaning of beer lines, often coupled with little attention to the tap room which should, of course, be to a good structural standard.

6) Unsuitable facilities for the preparation of bar foods. Sandwiches, soups and other bar snacks are in no way immune from being potential sources of food poisoning. They must be treated and prepared in the same way that they would be in any catering establishment. Adequate refrigeration and separate suitable preparation worktops are essential requirements. It is not acceptable to prepare any food for a commercial business in a domestic kitchen.

Common Problems in the Home

Your home may not be inspectable by the local Environmental Health Officer but it is still, nevertheless, a place where food is prepared. As many people suffer food poisoning from 'family' outbreaks, it is worthwhile to examine common factors which may contribute to these outbreaks.

1) Babies' nappies are often changed in unsuitable locations varying from the kitchen table to the settee. Nappies should be changed only on proper changing mats, the nappy being suitably and immediately disposed of. Other children should be kept way from the baby being changed and the hands of the changer should be scrubbed carefully in a wash-hand basin using soap and a nailbrush (never in the kitchen sink). The changing mat should be cleaned properly if it becomes soiled and it should be stored away carefully before the next use.

   Babies' bottles should not be kept in changing bags which may also contain wipes and creams, the containers of which are often handled by soiled hands during nappy changing.

2) Younger children should be supervised in hand-washing after using the toilet.

3) Dish-drying cloths should not be used as hand towels or wipe cloths and should be carefully stored between use - not on the back of a chair or indeed on the floor.

4) Many fridges are either not used sufficiently or do not store food at the correct temperature. Purchase a small fridge thermometer to check your fridge.

5) Family pets such as dogs and cats are often allowed free access to food storage and preparation areas, resulting in food contamination. Many pet lovers are oblivious to the fact that no matter how cuddly their pet may be, it may still carry disease-causing germs. Handwashing after handling pets is essential before food preparation or eating.

6) In farming households, insufficient attention may be given to the separation of the farming activities and those of the household, including child rearing. Because farmers must of necessity come in direct contact with animals, animal

slurries and frequently indirect contact with rodents on the farm, it is essential that the farmer practises good hygiene.

An outbuilding or garage should be designated as a changing area where dirty overalls, wellingtons or other footwear are removed.

This area should also be provided with good handwashing and drying facilities which should be used each time before re-entering the house. Access to the farmyard and sheds by children should be discouraged as much as possible and when this is not possible the same routine of wearing protective clothing and handwashing should be practised as already outlined.

7) Farming households often rely on raw milk instead of pasteurised milk.

While it seems foolish from an economic viewpoint to buy pasteurised milk, it is most important from a health standpoint, especially where the household includes children, elderly people or those who are ill.

8) The wipe cloth traditionally left by the kitchen sink should not be used to mop up spilled milk, to wipe the baby's face, or wipe food off the floor. Such cloths should be used only for very specific purposes and must be regularly changed and laundered.

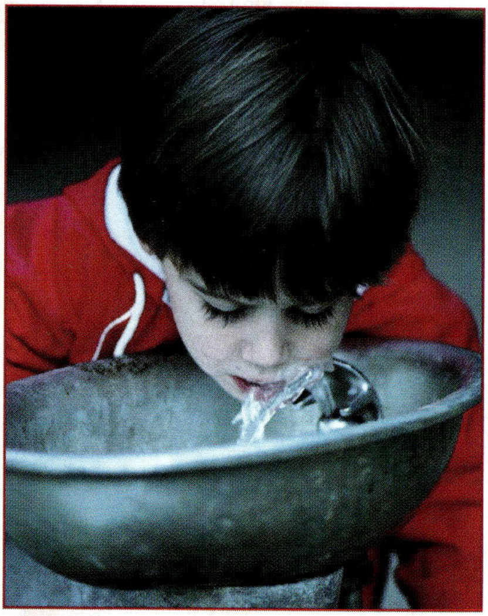

Always check that the water you use for drinking, food preparation, and ice-making is from an approved source and the supply is taken directly from the rising mains. If you are not sure of the quality of the water supplied to your premises have it analysed by the local Health Board.